Problems in
Arthritis and Rheumatism

Problems in Practice Series

Problems in Practice Series

Series Editors : J.Fry K.Williams M.Lancaster-Smith

Problems
in
Arthritis and
Rheumatism

Douglas N. Golding
MA MD FRCPI

Consultant Rheumatologist
Princess Alexandra Hospital, Harlow, Essex
and East Herts/West Essex Hospitals

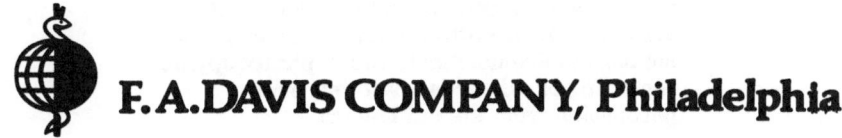

F.A.DAVIS COMPANY, Philadelphia

Published in North America by
F. A. Davis Company
1915 Arch Street
Philadelphia, PA 19103

Published in UK by
MTP Press Limited
Falcon House
Lancaster, England

First published 1981

LCCN 81 68109

ISBN-13: 978-94-009-8059-4   e-ISBN-13: 978-94-009-8057-0
DOI: 10.1007/ 978-94-009-8057-0

Contents

Contents

Series Foreword

This series of books is designed to help general practitioners. So are other books. What is unusual in this instance is their collective authorship; they are written by specialists working at district general hospitals. The writers derive their own experience from a range of cases less highly selected than those on which textbooks are traditionally based. They are also in a good position to pick out topics which they see creating difficulties for the practitioners of their district, whose personal capacities are familiar to them; and to concentrate on contexts where mistakes are most likely to occur. They are all well-accustomed to working in consultation.

All the authors write from hospital experience and from the viewpoint of their specialty. There are, therefore, matters important to family practice which should be sought not within this series, but elsewhere. Within the series much practical and useful advice is to be found with which the general practitioner can compare his existing performance and build in new ideas and improved techniques.

These books are attractively produced and I recommend them.

J. P. Horder OBE
President, The Royal College
of General Practitioners

SECTION 1
General Aspects

1 Introduction

Importance in practice – Classification of rheumatic disorders – Frequency of rheumatic disorders – Outcome and prognosis of rheumatic diseases

The importance of rheumatology in practice

'To the general practitioner, rheumatism may be just something of which he knows and understands little and for which he is prepared to just dole out a bottle of medicine or prescribe a liniment'. This was written 30 years ago by a celebrated rheumatologist of his time, Dr Francis Bach. The understanding of rheumatology by the family doctor has advanced a great deal since then: he knows how important it is to recognize the various types of rheumatism and arthritis and how effective proper treatment can be. Bottles of medicine and liniments have given way to carefully prescribed anti-inflammatory drugs and local steroid injections. The specialty of rheumatology has blossomed and has become infinitely more 'respectable' than it was, working in collaboration with orthopaedic surgery as well as with the various paramedical disciplines – physiotherapy, manipulation, occupational therapy and rehabilitation.

Diagnosis by the family doctor

For the family practitioner, four instances come to mind where it is particularly useful to be able to recognize and treat rheumatic conditions. Firstly, types of soft-tissue (non-articular) rheumatism are painful and distressing and may make work

Tennis elbow difficult or even impossible. An example is the common tennis elbow, which can be an extremely painful condition, but can often be rapidly cured by a properly placed local steroid injection. However, assuming that the injection is given correctly, should it not succeed in relieving pain there aré other possibilities – the pain may be referred to the elbow from an event in the cervical spine. Sometimes the advice of a rheumatologist is needed to sort out such tricky cases. Again, in the case of an inflammatory arthritis the precise diagnosis (rheumatoid arthritis, ankylosing spondylitis, gout) is essential for correct treatment. Rheumatism or arthritis can be the presenting feature of a systemic illness – for example, it may come as a surprise that polymyositis presenting with aching and weakness of the arms and legs may be 'secondary' to a malignant tumour somewhere, and pain and swelling of the wrist due to hypertrophic osteoarthropathy may be a feature of bronchogenic carcinoma. Finally, arthritis or rheumatism, though apparently the predominant symptom, can be just one feature of a systemic disorder, for example ulcerative colitis, hypothyroidism and sarcoidosis.

Psychosomatic rheumatism

As well as these possibilities the family doctor has to face a number of patients who persistently complain of 'rheumatism' yet seem to have little reason to do so. Many of these patients are elderly and often their symptoms relate to anxiety, depression, loneliness and despair. Should they be referred for specialist opinion, and if so, should they see a rheumatologist, a geriatrician, or perhaps a psychiatrist? Should they indeed be encouraged to be regular hospital attenders? At the same time

Possibilities of organic disease the practitioner must bear in mind that some organic illness may be lurking in the background. Is hypothyroidism being overlooked? Are those spasms of pain in the knees which appear clinically normal perhaps due to deposition of calcium crystals, in other words, is this chondrocalcinosis (pseudogout)? Could the aching, weak legs of a rheumatoid patient be due to spinal cord compression from atlanto-axial subluxation and not arthritis of the lower limb joints? Hospital investigation and a consultant opinion may be required to sort out such matters.

Less common conditions

This book attempts to highlight common problems of diagnosis and treatment of the rheumatic diseases as seen by the family physician. Attention is paid to those conditions commonly seen in practice and to some less common but nevertheless important rheumatic disorders, the rare and curious being mentioned only in passing. Such conditions as the Lesch–Nyhan syndrome (a very rare form of gout in children who have mental deficiency and certain neurological manifestations) are of interest to rheumatologists, who see in their elucidation a step towards the understanding of basic processes (in this particular case the absence of the enzyme HGPRT – hypoxanthine guanine phosphoribosyltransferase). Such conditions have little importance to the family doctor, who must nevertheless recognize or suspect that something is not quite as expected, and seek the advice of a rheumatologist – for instance the woman with rheumatoid arthritis who continues to lose weight and has marked anaemia and leukopenia may in fact suffer from Felty's syndrome or perhaps systemic lupus erythematosus; the young man who injured his back and was thought to have a mechanical lesion of the spine may turn out to have early ankylosing spondylitis. When the diagnosis is not straightforward the practitioner cannot always be expected to get it right, and throughout this book the indications for specialist referral have been given where relevant.

Rheumatism and arthritis as symptoms of other conditions

The classification of rheumatic disorders
Classification of arthritis

The classification of arthritis and rheumatism is far from adequate. Broadly speaking arthritis is either degenerative, traumatic, inflammatory, due to hypersensitivity (allergy) or secondary to some underlying condition. Degenerative arthritis (osteoarthritis or osteoarthrosis) is either 'primary', when it may involve many joints or just a few, or 'secondary' to an injury or previous inflammatory arthritis. Swelling of a joint after trauma (traumatic arthritis) is usually straightforward, but it must be remembered that the first symptoms of inflammatory or other types of joint disease may be precipitated by injury to the joint. Most cases of inflammatory arthritis fall into the category of rheumatoid disease but it is important to recognize the large variety of conditions which masquerade as this condition. Hypersensitivity arthritis may also resemble rheumatoid arthritis but can usually be associated with a drug reaction or other allergy. Arthritis secondary to another underlying disorder again may simulate rheumatoid or it may have specific features of its own – for instance, hypertrophic pulmonary osteoarthropathy, with its characteristic radiological features, which is

Degenerative arthritis

Traumatic arthritis

Inflammatory arthritis

Hypersensitivity arthritis

usually a manifestation of pulmonary neoplasm.

Inflammatory arthritis is either 'typical' rheumatoid arthritis (seropositive polyarthritis with erosive radiological changes) or an 'atypical' arthritis, that is one differing in several ways from typical rheumatoid. Atypical arthritis may be one of

Table 1.1   Atypical inflammatory arthritis

1. Atypical rheumatoid arthritis	joints not symmetrically involved; different joints (that is, only large joints) involved, atypical X-ray changes; persistently absent rheumatoid factor (seronegative)
2. Systemic connective tissue disease (such as systemic lupus erythematosus (SLE) polyarteritis, systemic sclerosis)	atypical joint involvement; high gammglobulin levels, circulating antibodies; immune complexes; high prevalence of systemic illness; specific associated lesions (such as skin or renal abnormalities); age and sex predilection; specific pathological changes
3. Seronegative spondarthritis	atypical peripheral arthritis; sacroiliitis or spondylitis; anterior uveitis (iritis); skin rashes (such as psoriasis); orogenital lesions, absent rheumatoid factor; presence of HLA B27
4. Infective arthritis	often monarthritis; acute onset with pyrexia; purulent synovial fluid containing organisms
5. Reactive (that is, post-infective) arthritis	latent period following focal infection (such as pharyngitis preceding rheumatic fever); transient or flitting arthritis of large joints; associated features (such as carditis in rheumatic fever, urethritis and conjunctivitis in Reiter's disease)
6. Metabolic arthritis (for example, gout)	usually acute onset in one or a few joints (classically MTP joint of big toe in gout); underlying metabolic abnormality (such as hyperuricaemia in gout)
7. Endocrine arthritis (for example, acromegalic arthritis)	atypical arthritis; endocrine abnormality
8. Arthritis of unknown origin (such as intermittent hydrarthrosis, Behçet's syndrome).	

several varieties, and the main distinguishing features of each are shown in Table 1.1.

Classification of rheumatism

The classification of rheumatism presents even more difficulty. It comprises a group of conditions often with vague or non-existent physical signs, implying anything from 'aches and pains' to specific, treatable conditions such as polymyalgia rheumatica. Many patients complaining of 'rheumatism' suffer from osteoarthritis of the spine or peripheral joints; often the pain can be traced to the cervical, thoracic or lumbar spine from which it is

Referred pain   referred. Indeed referred pain is probably the commonest type of rheumatism and its treatment is primarily that of the spinal lesion. Often, apparent 'soft-tissue rheumatism' appears to be associated with spinal lesions – for example, a supraspinatus lesion of the shoulder often coexists with cervical spondylosis. It seems that a spinal lesion not only refers pain to the limb but in some way it can 'set up' a local reaction, a focus of inflammation, such as a supraspinatus lesion or trochanteric bursitis. On the other hand there are specific varieties of soft tissue (non-articular) rheumatism, such as capsulitis of the shoulder and plantar fasciitis which seem to be definite entities. Under the heading of rheumatism we may also include myopathy, which may present with stiffness and aching rather than muscle weakness, though polymyositis and polymyalgia rheumatica are perhaps better included under the systemic connective tissue disorders. Polymyalgia is of course an important and common disorder (which is described in Chapter 12 under 'shoulder pain'). Finally, rheumatism covers the diffuse pains associated with certain chronic infections (such as brucellosis), metabolic disorders (such as osteomalacia), endocrine disorders (such as hypothyroidism), bone diseases (such as tumours and Paget's disease of bone) and certain hereditary disorders of connective tissue (for example the hypermobility syndrome).

The frequency of rheumatic disorders in family practice

Disorders of the musculoskeletal system comprise about 5 to 15% of cases seen in practice, that is, roughly one case in every ten coming to the surgery. An average family doctor would deal with 600 to 700 cases of 'rheumatism' each year. The prevalence of rheumatism is probably even higher than this if one takes into consideration the various types and gradations of severity of 'psychogenic' pain (see Chapter 4). Obviously, symptomatic osteoarthritis will turn up more often where there are a large number of elderly patients. Rheumatoid arthritis is much less common, but clearly has far-reaching importance with regard to prognosis and treatment (see Chapter 8).

Inherited disorders associated with rheumatism (such as Marfan's syndrome) are rare, but pain due to joint hypermobility is probably much less so. Gout occurs in only 0.3% but the incidence rises to 6% in first-degree relatives. Ankylosing spondylitis occurs in 0.1%, the incidence rising to 4% in first-degree relatives. The frequency of rheumatoid arthritis is about 1%, juvenile chronic arthritis (JCA) 0.05% in children under 15 years of age. With regard to osteoarthritis, moderate or severe radiological changes are seen in the hands of 11% of patients and in the hips of 0.5%, but radiological changes do not necessarily relate to symptoms (see Chapter 3). The painful shoulder occurs in 16% and tennis elbow in 3% of patients attending the surgery. The average prevalence of polymyalgia rheumatica is 0.04% but this rises to 0.8% in the over-80s. Rheumatic disorders account for 10% of working days lost.

In conclusion, the general practitioner sees one to three new cases of rheumatic disease every day. Most can be managed without specialist help, and indeed fewer cases of 'rheumatism' are referred to hospital than in other specialities. Practitioners should have a sound idea of the reasons and indication for referral for specialist advice, and this important topic is covered in detail in Chapter 3.

The outcome and prognosis of rheumatic diseases

When a patient is told that he has rheumatoid arthritis he is particularly concerned with the prognosis – his own particular prognosis. He gets little comfort from being told that accurate prediction of the outcome is difficult if not impossible. Nevertheless the physician should be in a position to let him know the *likely* sequel of events and the *approximate* chance of severe disability (Table 1.2).

Table 1.2 Factors linked to prognosis in rheumatoid arthritis

1. Mode of onset	acute onset of polyarthritis is usually favourable
2. Sex	generally males tend to do better than females
3. Age	onset in later life is favourable

Table 1.2 (Cont'd)

4. Initial joint involvement	a monarticular, asymmetrical onset is favourable
5. Initial erythrocyte sedimentation rate (ESR)	a high ESR at the onset is unfavourable
6. The X-ray	a persistently normal X-ray is a good sign; erosive changes seen at an early stage is unfavourable
7. Rheumatoid factor	persistently seronegative cases do better than cases which are seropositive from the onset (other features peculiar to seropositive cases, such as subcutaneous nodules and vasculitis, are also indicative of a poor prognosis)

Soft-tissue lesions

Most soft-tissue (non-articular) types of rheumatism (such as tennis elbow, plantar fasciitis, rotator cuff lesions of the shoulder) have a self-limiting course which can be shortened and made more comfortable by correct treatment. Sometimes the condition is stubborn, and here it is often the case that either (a) the treatment has been incorrect or imprecise, or (b) there is some underlying factor, hitherto unrecognized (such as referred pain from the spine being responsible for persistent tennis elbow). It is important to recognize that certain soft-tissue conditions have a protracted course, the best example being the frozen shoulder (capsulitis) which takes many months to resolve (see Chapter 12).

Osteoarthritis

A 'worn-down' joint obviously cannot be 'cured' (though it may be possible to replace it by a prosthesis, as in total hip replacement). However, the patient should be reassured that in the great majority of cases symptoms will settle down, deformity is unlikely and disability very unusual. There are exceptions – osteoarthritis of the hip has a 60–70% chance of steadily getting worse until movements become grossly restricted as well as painful, when surgery is required. When osteoarthritis occurs after a previous injury, such as a fracture, it has less chance of settling down quickly than primary osteoarthritis. Severe osteoarthritis of the knees can lead to progressive loss of cartilage in the medial or lateral compartments, resulting in genu valgum or varus with their consequent mechanical effects on the knee joint and therefore on mobility.

Rheumatoid arthritis

It has been mentioned how difficult it is to predict the outcome in a newly diagnosed patient with rheumatoid arthritis. Nevertheless, reassurance should be couched in the following terms:

30% of cases do quite well: pain and stiffness is well controlled by suitable treatment, deformities do not occur or are only slight. Most if not all the usual activities of daily living remain possible.

50% of cases do well

20% of cases do very well indeed: these are long remissions, and only occasionally are analgesic tablets for pain relief required. The quality of life is hardly affected.

40% of cases are progressive, needing constant medical supervision, although pain and disability can be minimized by proper treatment; at least some degree of deformity is likely in this group.

50% of cases do not do so well

Only 10% of cases progress relentlessly, with severe deformities and consequent marked disability. Serious complications are most likely in this group.

Ankylosing spondylitis

The outcome of ankylosing spondylitis is greatly improved when proper treatment (such as anti-inflammatory drugs and exercise therapy) is instituted at an early stage, thereby preventing postural deformity and possibly diminishing the likelihood of severe restriction of spinal movements. Females apparently are much less likely to develop severe spinal stiffness, and spondylitis in general is milder in women. The prognostically poor features in ankylosing spondylitis are:

(1) Progressive involvement of the hips.
(2) Severe involvement of the cervical spine leading to severe restriction of neck movements and sometimes atlanto-axial subluxation.
(3) Severe involvement of the thoracic spine leading to respiratory disability.
(4) Systemic complications such as uveitis, aortic valve disease or amyloidosis.
(5) A very high ESR, wasting and constitutional disability.

20

Introduction

Gout

The whole conception of gout including prognosis has been completely transformed by the introduction of drugs which lower the body's uric acid. When attacks of gout are allowed to continue and hyperuricaemia is not controlled chronic gouty arthritis, tophi and progressive renal insufficiency are likely. The prescription of uric acid lowering drugs (particularly allopurinol) leads to the diminution of frequency and severity of acute attacks, often abolishing them altogether, and makes complications extremely unlikely.

2 Some illustrative problems

Ankylosing spondylitis – Non-steroidal anti-inflammatory drugs – Pain and paraesthesiae in arms – The acute back – The painful foot – A gouty attack – The painful hip – A knee effusion – Laboratory investigations – The acute neck – Helpful organizations – Polymyalgia rheumatica – Early rheumatoid arthritis – The painful shoulder – Tennis elbow

This book is about problems of arthritis and rheumatism as encountered in practice. Examples of such problems given here are by way of introduction to the text, which should be consulted where relevant – as indicated by the reference chapter given at the end of each problem.

Ankylosing spondylitis: its early diagnosis in a young man with backache

Suspicion of ankylosing spondylitis may be aroused when pain affects several parts of the spine and perhaps the anterior thoracic region, causing a feeling of breathlessness. The back is stiff in the morning for perhaps some hours. Movements of the spine are limited in many directions (rather than in just one or two places) and chest expansion may be reduced. The ESR may be raised, but not necessarily so. Radiographs of the spine and sacro-iliac joints may show some abnormality in early cases, but this is not always clear and in these circumstances referral for consultant opinion may be wise – do not rely too heavily on the X-ray report! (See Chapter 9.)

23

(Non-steroidal) anti-inflammatory drugs – which to use?

The number and variety of available anti-inflammatory drugs is legion. It is helpful to remember that:

(1) Patients often respond differently to different anti-inflammatory drugs.
(2) Side-effects occur in some patients and not in others.
(3) These drugs often lose their effect after some time, when a change may be indicated.
(4) A night dose often relieves early morning stiffness.
(5) If possible, once-daily (or evening) dosage is convenient and may be sufficient.
(6) Avoid all anti-inflammatory drugs if there is a current or recent peptic ulcer. Only paracetamol (or perhaps benorylate) may be given by mouth, but others may be cautiously tried in the form of suppositories.
(7) Other precautions to heed are: pregnancy, concomitant anti-coagulant therapy and renal or hepatic dysfunction. (See Chapter 5.)

Pain and paraesthesiae in arms – what causes it?

This may be due to a neck problem (such as a disc lesion) or a carpal tunnel syndrome – but sometimes *both* operate! Both lesions, if present, require treatment in their own right. This requires careful elucidation of the diagnosis, often requiring special investigations such as electrodiagnosis. (See Chapter 12.)

The acute back – what to do?

It may or may not be possible to say whether an attack of acute back pain is due to a prolapsed disc, simply a back strain or intervertebral joint derangement. In any event, complete rest and the prescription of analgesics and muscle relaxants are correct initial therapy. If the pain has not resolved within 2 or 3 days a decision must be made as to whether a further period of complete bed-rest, perhaps in hospital, is advisable, or alternatively mobilization (by manipulation or physiotherapy) is required. Sciatica gradually coming on after backache usually implies a progressive disc lesion and here complete rest is essential. Conversely, a 'stuck back' with no symptoms or signs in the legs usually implies a mechanical joint derangement which often responds to manipulation. (See Chapter 11.)

The painful foot – what might it be?

The pain may be simply due to chronic foot strain, as from pes planus or cavus. However, it must be remembered that rheumatoid arthritis often presents with pain in the 'balls of the feet' (metatarsophalangeal joints), which are tender when squeezed. Really severe, acute pain in the foot might be due to a stress fracture of one of the small bones, or perhaps an attack of gout. (See Chapter 13.)

A gouty attack –which drugs to use?

The acute attack of gout is best 'smashed on the head' by a large dose of one of the non-steroidal anti-inflammatory drugs, such as phenylbutazone or indomethacin, for a day or two, which is then tailed off. Even though the serum uric acid be raised, it is important that allopurinol is *not* given at this stage. After the attack has subsided, if the serum uric acid is consistently high, then prescribe allopurinol to get the S.U.A. down, in order to prevent future attacks of gout. (See Chapter 10.)

The painful hip –what to do?

First, decide whether the pain *is* coming from the hip joint (usually osteoarthritis), or perhaps referred from a spinal lesion – usually an upper lumbar disc or area of spondylosis. X-rays of the lumbar spine and pelvis are usually required. Spinal referred pain will often respond to physiotherapy or perhaps acupuncture. Osteoarthritis of the hip will often require surgery if it is at all severe or progressive. However, the pain may arise from the hip and also *aggravated* by referred pain from the spine – so it is always worth treating this, if present, even if the X-ray shows osteoarthritic changes in the hip. (See Chapter 13.)

A knee effusion – what to do?

A persistent effusion in the knee should always be *aspirated*. This gives relief of pain as well as diagnostic information. If the fluid is turbid it should be sent for culture and examination for cells and crystals. (See Chapters 3, 5 and 13.)

Laboratory investigations – which are most helpful in the diagnosis of arthritis?

From a practical point of view the most useful investigations are:

(1) Full blood count and ESR (which is nearly always raised in inflammatory arthritis and connective tissue disease).
(2) Test for rheumatoid factor.
(3) Serum uric acid (the blood urea/creatinine should always be requested at the time, as hyperuricaemia may occur in renal dysfunction).
(4) Urine test for albumin and blood.
(5) Synovial fluid analysis, when obtained from joint effusions. (See Chapter 3.)

The acute neck – what to do?

Arrange for a soft collar and prescribe adequate analgesics and muscle relaxants. An X-ray does not usually give useful information (unless the patient is known to have rheumatoid arthritis, when, for example atlanto-axial subluxation may be seen). Should the pain fail to settle after a day or two physiotherapy may be indicated. Sometimes a manipulation will correct an acute intervertebral joint derangement ('locked joint'), but this should not be attempted where there is clear evidence of a prolapsed cervical disc or impending disc lesion as shown by brachial neuralgia and paraesthesiae in the arm.

Helpful organizations for the arthritic patient

The A.R.C. and B.R.A. are two. The Arthritis and Rheumatism Council (8–10 Charing Cross Rd., London) is mainly concerned with research, but provides help to patients such as the provision of handbooks on various conditions (which can be purchased by post). The British Rheumatism and Arthritis Association (B.R.A.), 6 Grosvenor Crescent, London, provides information on arthritis and practical aids.

Polymyalgia rheumatica – how to recognize it?

It must be realized that this is not just a name given to describe vague aches and pains in the back and limbs. Polymyalgia is a distinct syndrome characterized by quite severe pain in the shoulders and hips, prolonged morning stiffness and a high ESR, usually in elderly patients. Exclusion of early rheumatoid arthritis, which may present in this way, is important. Sometimes polymyalgia is secondary to temporal arteritis – a temporal artery biopsy is sometimes (though not always) indicated. The response to steroids is usually brisk, and failure to respond immediately should cast doubt on the diagnosis. (See Chapter 6.)

Early rheumatoid arthritis – can we give a firm prognosis?

Unfortunately, the simple answer is – no. However, there are some factors linked to prognosis, such as mode of onset (whether acute or gradual), the number of joints involved at the onset and whether rheumatoid factor is present at an early stage. If bone erosions are seen in the X-ray soon after the onset the outcome will probably be less favourable than in cases which remain 'non-erosive' for the first year or two. (See Chapter 1.)

Sorting out the painful shoulder

Shoulder pain is often a problem and it is important to come to a diagnosis. In most cases the pain is either referred from a cervical spine lesion, or else due to a soft-tissue lesion around the shoulder – usually a rotator cuff lesion or capsulitis (frozen shoulder). Patients are worried about the possibility of shoulder arthritis – they can be firmly reassured that this is rare. In rotator cuff lesions (such as supraspinatus tendinitis), the shoulder movements are painful but full. In capsulitis (frozen shoulder), movements are limited in all directions, recovery is protracted but treatment is beneficial. (See Chapter 12.)

The stubborn tennis elbow

Usually, but not always, the common tennis elbow responds to a *correctly-placed* local steroid injection. Cases unresponsive to one or two local steroid injections are usually 'secondary' to some other underlying condition such as cervical spondylosis (referring pain into the arm) or osteoarthritis of the elbow. It will be clear that treatment of any underlying condition, as well as local treatment of the tennis elbow, is indicated. (See Chapter 12).

3 Diagnosis and assessment of rheumatic disorders

Symptoms, signs and their diagnostic significance – X-rays and laboratory investigations – Early diagnosis: indications for referral

Correct diagnosis depends on the interpretation of presenting symptoms and signs together with laboratory and radiological investigations. Perhaps especially in rheumatic disorders treatment cannot be usefully applied until a correct diagnosis is made, though symptomatic measures are sometimes possible before definite diagnosis.

Symptoms, signs and their diagnostic significance

The symptoms and signs of rheumatism and arthritis are (a) those related to the joints and musculoskeletal structures (articular symptoms and signs), and (b) those arising outside the musculoskeletal system (non-articular symptoms and signs).

Articular symptoms and signs

These are: pain, stiffness, swelling, tenderness, limited movements, deformity, paraesthesiae, muscle wasting and weakness.

Pain

Joint pain   Joint pain is the cardinal symptom of arthritis (though pain in or around the joints may also occur in soft-tissue and various forms

29

of non-articular rheumatism). In arthritis, pain at rest nearly always denotes active inflammation of the joint, usually synovitis. Pain induced by weight-bearing or movement may be due to involvement of other structures in the joint, such as cartilage erosion, or fraying or inflammation of the ligaments in osteoarthritis (ligamentous strain pain). On the other hand, pain may be entirely mechanical and not due to active inflammation when there are abnormal strains and stresses on the joint, such as in genu varum or valgum, or flattening of the arches of the feet. Again, pain may not come from the joint or other local structures. It is often *referred* from the spine or elsewhere and the recognition of referred pain is of paramount importance in rheumatology, as it can often mimic arthritis. For example, pain in the knuckles (in the absence of swelling) may be referred in a patient with cervical spondylosis; the metacarpophalangeal joints may even be tender on palpation. Such referred pain is recognized after local arthritis has been excluded clinically and by appropriate investigations, and evidence of cervical root involvement (such as an absent deep reflex or corresponding diminution of sensation as well as local signs in the neck) is found. Again, when pain is described as 'burning' or 'stabbing' suspicion may be aroused that the pain is not organic but part of an anxiety or depressive state. When due to compression of a nerve-root leaving the spine, sciatica or brachial neuralgia is nearly always accompanied by paraesthesiae in the corresponding dermatomes. However, pain can be simply referred down a limb from a spinal lesion and then there are no accompanying paraesthesiae.

Ligamentous strain pain *(margin note)*

Referred pain *(margin note)*

Stiffness

Joint stiffness *(margin note)*

'Stiffness' may relate to either the joints or muscles. Joint stiffness is either due to *inflammation*, when it is felt at rest and most severe in the morning, or *mechanical*, when the stiffness occurs on moving the joint and is due to pathological changes within it. Muscle stiffness may be *physiological*, as after strenuous exercise; *inflammatory*, as in polymyositis; or *apparent* – patients often say that a weak limb feels 'stiff'.

Muscle stiffness *(margin note)*

Swelling

Joint swelling *(margin note)*

Pain is the cardinal symptom, and joint swelling the cardinal sign of arthritis. It is important to note that patients often say a joint or limb feels swollen but examination does not reveal

30

Diagnosis and assessment

swelling and, on questioning, actual enlargement of the part has not been noticed, or is admitted to be very slight. To be certain the physician should *observe* swelling on at least one occasion. This may be actual swelling of the joint, swelling of structures related to the joint (such as bursitis or tenosynovitis) or swelling of structures away from the joint (such as fat deposits in panniculitis). Joint swelling is usually due to synovial hypertrophy (synovitis) with or without an effusion. Effusions can often be diagnosed clinically and proof is provided by aspiration of synovial fluid, which can provide useful diagnostic information.

Joint effusions

Tenderness

Joint tenderness

Pressure on an inflamed joint produces tenderness. Inflamed soft tissue is also tender to palpation and this is often the principal, or only, evidence in soft-tissue lesions such as epicondylitis (tennis and golfer's elbows), supraspinatus tendinitis and plantar fasciitis. In spinal lesions, even though a patient has normal back movements local tenderness over one or more vertebrae may isolate the spinal abnormality. Tenderness is therefore an extremely important physical sign in rheumatology, being of great localizing value in many cases, though again the possibility of 'referred tenderness' (mentioned above) must be borne in mind.

Limitation of movements

Stiffness is a symptom, and objective limitation of movements a physical sign. A hip may feel stiff but on examination it moves fully: more than likely the trouble is referred from the upper lumbar spine and not due to hip-joint disease. A stiff shoulder in which there is a full range of passive movements is probably a rotator cuff lesion, while limitation of abduction and rotation denotes capsulitis (frozen shoulder). Movements may be limited by muscle spasm, when it is difficult to say whether there is an objective cause for the restriction, one example being the patient with cervical spondylosis and a superimposed 'whiplash' injury precipitated by a road traffic accident. It is sometimes possible to clarify this by abolishing the muscle spasm through injecting relaxants such as diazepam, or by needling an acupuncture point.

Frozen shoulder

Deformity

While slight degrees of ulnar deviation are sometimes seen in early cases of rheumatoid arthritis, generally speaking

31

deformity is not an early feature of any kind of arthritis. Acute spinal disorders, such as cervical or lumbar disc lesions and intervertebral joint derangements, may present with torticollis or scoliosis. Patients with early ankylosing spondylitis sometimes tend to be round-shouldered, but this posture is assumed in order to relieve pain and can be corrected by postural training and exercises – unlike structural deformity such as the permanent kyphosis seen in advanced stages of the disease. In rheumatoid arthritis classical established deformities, such as ulnar deviation or swan-neck deformities of the fingers, are often diagnostic.

Paraesthesiae

Pins-and-needles, numbness or tingling in a limb usually denote either compression of a nerve-root or inflammation of a nerve (neuritis). It must be remembered that pressure on a nerve at more than one level may summate to produce symptoms – for example, paraesthesiae in the outside of the arm and thumb may be due to a combination of a 5th cervical disc lesion and a carpal tunnel syndrome – and each of these may require treatment in its own right. Paraesthesiae are occasionally encountered in multiple sclerosis, in peripheral vascular disorders and in peripheral neuritis (where the paraesthesiae are felt in all four limbs). Usually pain and paraesthesia in the same dermatome implies a compressive lesion of the same nerve root, as in sciatica due to S_1 root compression by a prolapsed lumbar disc.

Muscle wasting and weakness

Muscle wasting

Apparent 'weakness' may really be the effect of pain in the joints. In arthritis and the connective tissue disorders, true muscle wasting may be due to several reasons. In persistent active arthritis there may be marked generalized wasting of flesh; should one joint remain 'active' the muscles acting on the joint – for example, the quadriceps muscles in persistent knee synovitis – will atrophy. Muscle wasting can be due to a true myopathy (muscle-wasting disorder), this being not uncommon in many of the systemic connective-tissue disorders as well as in rheumatoid disease (in dermatomyositis and polymyositis muscle wasting and weakness is, of course, the cardinal feature).

Steroid myopathy

Certain anti-inflammatory drugs, in particular systemic steroids, can produce a myopathy – the steroids with a halogen in the molecule, particularly triamcinolone (now rarely used in arthritis) were especially likely to do so.

Diagnosis and assessment

Non-articular symptoms and signs

These may be related to mental state, or to disorders of the skin and nails, blood vessels, eyes, cardiorespiratory system, kidneys, blood, spleen and lymph nodes.

Skin and nail disorders

The skin and nails can give useful clues in the early diagnosis of many types of rheumatic and connective tissue disease. Some examples are as follows:

(1) *Systemic connective tissue diseases* – the thick, hide-bound skin of systemic sclerosis, the typical rash in the 'butterfly' region of the face in systemic lupus, livido reticularis in polyarteritis.
(2) *Skin lesions in specific arthropathies* – typical skin and nail lesions in psoriatic arthritis, Reiter's disease and Behçet's disease.
(3) *Erythema nodosum* as an initial feature of sarcoidosis, focal streptococcal infection or ulcerative colitis – all of which may be associated with some form of arthritis or rheumatism.

Vascular disorders

Arteritis

Vasodilatation is of course one of the cardinal features of the inflammatory reaction and therefore of all types of inflammatory arthritis. Vascular lesions of clinical significance in arthritis and connective tissue disorders are due to a specific inflammation of the arterial wall called arteritis, which can have local effects, such as skin infarcts or ulcers, and more serious generalized effects. Widespread arteritis is a complication of some severe cases of rheumatoid arthritis, but it may occur at an early stage in other connective tissue disorders such as polyarteritis. Arteritis does not occur in gout and is very rare in ankylosing spondylitis. In early cases of rheumatoid arthritis tiny haemorrhages in the finger-pulps and nail-folds due to a more benign form of vascular lesion may be seen.

Eye disorders

Useful information may be gleaned by examination of the eye. Perhaps best-known is iridocyclitis (anterior uveitis) associated with ankylosing spondylitis where it is often an early feature, or may even precede back pain, scleritis, episcleritis or dry eyes (keratoconjunctivitis sicca) in early rheumatoid disease, conjunctivitis (a cardinal feature of Reiter's disease), and other types of eye inflammation seen in certain less common conditions such as Behçet's syndrome.

Respiratory disorders

Pleurisy (wet or dry) or pericarditis may be early features in rheumatoid disease. Various cardiac and pulmonary lesions occur in many systemic connective-tissue disorders (see the Glossary at the end of this book), though they are not usually of diagnostic importance in the early stages. In ankylosing spondylitis involvement of the costovertebral and sternomanubrial joints may make breathing difficult. (In late cases of spondylitis restriction of chest expansion may lead to recurrent pneumonitis and a specific type of upper lobe fibrosis.) Conversely, certain rheumatic syndromes (for example, hypertrophic osteoarthropathy and capsulitis of the shoulders) may be a premonitory feature of serious pulmonary disease such as neoplasm.

Renal disorders

Albuminuria The discovery of albuminuria on routine urine testing often means a simple urinary infection, but otherwise may indicate glomerular dysfunction as a result of a connective tissue disorder such as polyarteritis and systemic lupus erythematosus (SLE). Except for the possibilities of chronic pyelonephritis and the rare complication of amyloid disease, renal disease is not a feature of rheumatoid arthritis (although a late feature of chronic gout). Chronic renal failure may be a clue to the diagnosis of osteomalacia which is an important cause of back pain, weakness and 'rheumatism' felt in the thighs and hips, because renal failure is one cause of this condition.

Blood disorders

Anaemia Pallor may indicate anaemia, an early feature of rheumatoid arthritis and some connective tissue disorders. Anaemia of any degree is unlikely in osteoarthritis, ankylosing spondylitis, gout or non-articular rheumatism. Anaemia may, of course, be aggravated by blood loss such as that due to gastrointestinal irritation by current antirheumatic drugs.

Lymphadenopathy

Small lymph nodes are sometimes felt in rheumatoid arthritis but multiple, large nodes are unusual, except in children (Still's disease) and in Felty's syndrome (see the glossary at the end of this book). Enlarged lymph glands are often found in active cases of systemic lupus erythematosus.

Splenomegaly

In rheumatology, a large spleen draws attention to the possibilities of Felty's syndrome, systemic lupus and juvenile polyarthritis. The spleen is of course enlarged in leukaemia (in which joint and musculoskeletal pain is common) and secondary gout may occur in these patients.

Psychological disorders

Nearly all patients presenting with rheumatism or arthritis are anxious, some are depressed, many are worried that they are on the brink of a crippling arthritis. All possible reassurance is most important. Early rheumatoid arthritis is often associated Anxiety with anxiety and this is particularly marked in menopausal and Depression premenopausal patients. Depression is an important feature of polymyalgia rheumatica and it responds dramatically to systemic steroids. More serious nervous problems and psychoses may occur in patients with systemic lupus erythematosus. It is common knowledge that a patient suffering from recurrent gout is irritable and 'difficult'. Finally, symptoms of rheumatism and arthritis are themselves frequently aggravated by anxiety and depressive states, as discussed in Chapter 4.

X-rays and laboratory investigations

In many patients presenting with rheumatic symptoms a diagnosis can be made without the need for special investigations, such as soft-tissue rheumatism or degenerative joint disease. This is not usually the case in acute or chronic arthritis or in apparently obscure cases of 'rheumatism', particularly if this is generalized; here X-rays and laboratory tests are often useful, though their correct interpretation is not always straightforward.

Table 3.1 Basic investigations in rheumatic disease

X-ray hands, feet, chest, spine and sacroiliac joints.
HB, WBC, ESR
Latex (or other test for rheumatoid factor)
ANA
SUA, blood urea, serum creatinine
Routine urinalysis (protein, blood, sugar)
Aspiration of synovial fluid (if effusion present)

Useful investigations in rheumatology are as follows (see also Table 3.1):

(1) X-ray examination of the joints and spine.
(2) Haematology, especially haemogloblin, white cell count and erythrocyte sedimentation rate (ESR).
(3) Immunology, especially tests for rheumatoid factor, anti-nuclear antibodies, DNA binding, HLA antigens and immunoelectrophoresis of plasma globulins.
(4) Blood chemistry, especially protein electrophoresis, serum uric acid, serum calcium, phosphorus and phosphatases and serum muscle enzymes.
(5) Urine tests, routine testing for albumin and blood, mid-stream specimen for cells and organisms.
(6) Synovial fluid, its appearance and viscosity, microscopic examination for cells, crystals and pathogenic organisms.

Biopsy

(Note: joint biopsy and arthroscopy are occasionally useful investigations carried out in hospital but not in general practice. Synovial biopsy can be useful in the diagnosis of tuberculous arthritis and occasionally in certain inflammatory arthropathies. Muscle biopsy may be useful in the diagnosis of myopathies, biopsy of skin nodules in doubtful cases of rheumatoid arthritis and in xanthomatosis, skin biopsy in systemic sclerosis, arterial biopsy in polyarteritis, temporal arteritis and

Arthroscopy

polymyalgia rheumatica. The main use of arthroscopy of the knee is to isolate meniscal lesions, but occasionally visualization of the synovium is helpful in elucidating doubtful monarthritis.)

X-ray examination of the joints and spine

There must always be clear reasons for requesting an X-ray. For example, in the case of a swollen knee joint it should be realized that X-rays often show nothing of significance, except in some instances such as crystal deposition disease. A much more useful procedure would be to aspirate the knee and examine the synovial fluid. On the other hand, in a patient with polyarthritis

X-rays in
back pain

X-rays of the hands and feet may give valuable evidence of early rheumatoid arthritis. There is controversy as to whether spinal X-rays should be carried out routinely in patients with a first attack of low back pain. X-rays give little information in a young patient with backache following direct or indirect injury. On the other hand, failure to X-ray the spine of an elderly patient with chronic back pain may lead to failure to diagnose a tumour or perhaps severe osteoporosis with crush fracture.

While in the early stages plain radiographs are often normal, Table 3.2 shows some examples of changes that can be very helpful in diagnosis:

Table 3.2

Rheumatoid arthritis	periarticular osteoporosis, small articular erosions, periosteal reaction
Osteoarthritis	narrowing of the joint space, osteophytes ('lipping'), para-articular sclerosis.
Ankylosing spondylitis	irregularity, narrowing or lack of definition ('fuzziness') of the sacroiliac joints; ankylosis of the spine and sacroiliac joints does not occur in early stages of this condition but sometimes vertebral erosions or syndesmophytes (spikes of bone vertically connecting two contiguous vertebra) may be seen in the X-ray
Gout	if a joint has been the site of several previous attacks small punched-out erosions or cysts may be seen.

Special X-rays

Use of
myelograms
and
arthrograms

Special types of X-ray examination, such as myelograms and arthrograms, are often useful tools for the rheumatologist and orthopaedic surgeon but not for the family physician. The following example illustrates this. A patient presenting with severe sciatica and weakness of the legs was found to have evidence of cord compression due to cervical spondylosis (cervical myelopathy) as well as a large lumbar disc lesion. The sciatic pain settled down with bedrest and traction, but walking remained difficult owing to the myelopathy causing leg weakness. Because the patient was elderly and had recently had several operations, some of which were followed by complications, it was not considered that an operation on the spine would be advisable in the near future so a myelogram was not ordered at the time.

Haematological investigations

Together with routine urinalysis, basic haematology – haemoglobin, white cell count and differential and erythrocyte sedimentation rate (ESR) – represents minimal investigation in rheumatic disorders and is essential in patients presenting with inflammatory polyarthritis. Early in this chapter the importance of anaemia was mentioned. The typical anaemia of rheumatoid arthritis (RA) is a normocytic, normochromic anaemia, the haemoglobin being around 10–12 g/dl. Leukocytosis occasionally occurs in rheumatoid disease but is not a typical feature – if marked, it should raise suspicion of a superadded infection (either systemic or a septic arthritis), a post-infective arthritis ('reactive') such as rheumatic fever, or one of the varieties of polyarteritis. Leukopenia occurs in systemic lupus erythematosus and in Felty's syndrome (for RA with hypersplenism, see the glossary at the end of this book) but the commonest cause of a low white cell count in a patient with RA is drug sensitivity, and many antirheumatic drugs (for example, phenylbutazone) may be responsible for this.

Anaemia in rheumatoid arthritis

Leukocytosis and leukopenia

Erythrocyte sedimentation rate (ESR)

The erythrocyte sedimentation rate (ESR) – the 'rheumatologists' yardstick' – is a useful pointer to inflammatory joint disease (and also to neoplastic disease, as for example when a raised ESR occurs in a patient with back pain.) The ESR is usually raised in rheumatoid arthritis, ankylosing spondylitis, acute gout, polymyalgia rheumatica, the systemic connective-tissue disorders and a variety of less common arthritic disorders such as Reiter's disease and infective arthritis. The ESR is *not* raised in degenerative or metabolic joint disease or in soft-tissue rheumatism. When an ESR is raised it should be repeated, especially if there is no apparent reason for its elevation. It can then be helpful to look at the serum globulins, immunoglobulins and acid and alkaline phosphatases. The Westergren method of estimating the ESR is now universally used. ESRs of up to 20 mm/hour (in males) and up to 25 mm/hour (in females) are accepted as within normal limits in rheumatology practice.

Raised ESR

Immunological investigations

Immunological tests are now standard in hospital diagnosis and the practitioner should familiarize himself with interpretation of the more basic tests. This is because inflammatory arthritis is usually associated with abnormalities of the immune system which basically includes (a) the cellular immune response (B and T cells), not a standard test in the laboratory; (b) abnormalities of the humeral response, that is, immunoglobulin antibodies, the detection of which is now routinely carried out by hospital laboratories; and (c) abnormalities of serum complement – occasionally useful, but which can be left to the rheumatologist for interpretation.

Rheumatoid factor (RF)

Rheumatoid factor (RF) is the most commonly requested immunological investigation. This is usually an IgM (immunoglobulin M) antibody in the serum which under certain circumstances reacts with altered IgG (immunoglobulin G) to form 'particles', or else with complement also to form 'immune complexes'. These complexes are thought to be the direct cause of certain characteristic phenomena of connective tissue disorders such as vasculitis and renal disease. Rheumatoid factor is found in the blood of 75% of patients with rheumatoid arthritis of more than 12 months duration, but in only 40–50% of those with early disease. Therefore *absence of rheumatoid factor does not preclude a diagnosis of RA*, and conversely this diagnosis should never be allowed to rest only on the presence of rheumatoid factor. Finally, RF is *not diagnostic* of rheumatoid arthritis as it can be found in other conditions such as liver disease, sarcoidosis, subacute bacterial endocarditis and in 4% of healthy adults. When there is a definite inflammatory arthritis and rheumatoid factor is persistently absent the arthritis is said to be *seronegative*. It may still turn out to be rheumatoid arthritis, but steps must now be taken to find out if the arthritis is in fact one of the varieties grouped under the heading of 'seronegative spondarthritis' (see Chapter 9) or else perhaps one of the connective tissue disorders which is often seronegative, such as polyarteritis. Essentially this means requesting antinuclear antibodies and HLA antigens (see below). Finally, there remain a group of seronegative inflammatory arthritis of uncertain nature, some of which respond to treatment like RA, whereas others do not and are a therapeutic enigma.

Rheumatoid factor is detected by one or more of the following tests: sheep-cell agglutination (Rose Waaler) test, latex agglutination test and RAHA test. It is important to note whether or not the result is *strongly* positive. The Rose Waaler test is

Rheumatoid factor in the blood

Tests for RF

given as a titre; below 1 : 32 is not significant, 1 : 64 is definitely positive and values above 1 : 500 are highly positive, usually indicating severe rheumatoid disease.

Antinuclear antibody (ANA)

ANA and DNA in SLE

Serum complement level

Antinuclear antibody (ANA) is present in all cases of systemic lupus erythematosus (SLE), but again it is not specific for this condition as it may appear in other connective tissue diseases such as systemic sclerosis, and occasionally (though in low titre) in rheumatoid arthritis. The ANA titre is important, and titres of 1 : 200 or more are likely to indicate SLE. Of more specific help in the diagnosis of SLE is the presence of antiDNA antibodies (DNA binding). LE cells occur in the blood of only 75% of cases of SLE and again may occasionally be found in rheumatoid arthritis. Therefore, in order to definitely prove the diagnosis of SLE, there should be negative rheumatoid factor, strongly positive ANA, raised DNA-binding and perhaps LE cells too. In this condition the level of serum complement is also useful, as it is low in active disease.

Immunoglobulins

Myeloma

Immunoglobulins can give useful information when the ESR is raised for no obvious reason. In seropositive rheumatoid arthritis serum IgM is usually (though not always) raised, representing rheumatoid factor in the blood. Otherwise there may be a polycolonal increase of all immunoglobulins, such as IgA, IgG and IgM. In rubella (with which arthritis may be associated) IgM is raised and here this represents rubella antibodies. IgA, synthesized in mucous membranes, may be raised in Sjogren's syndrome, where exocrine secretions are deficient. The immunoglobulin profile can show the abnormal paraprotein found in myelomatosis which can present in rheumatology departments with joint pain, backache, polymyalgia or secondary amyloid disease. The immunoglobulins are absent or deficient in the rare condition hypogammaglobinaemia (congenital or acquired), with which a form of arthritis may be associated.

The Wassermann reaction (WR) and gonococcal complement fixation test (GCFT)

WR
GCFT

In rheumatology departments these tests are usually requested in patients suspected as having Reiter's syndrome. However, a positive GCFT is only rarely found in this condition. This test is of more importance where gonococcal arthritis is common, such as in the United States.

The antistreptolysis O titre (ASO)

ASO   This is made to detect focal streptococcal infection and is of course essential in the diagnosis of rheumatic fever, now a very rare condition. It is uncertain as to whether 'benign' forms of rheumatic fever ('subacute rheumatism') associated with a high ASO exist – many later turn out to be cases of rheumatoid arthritis.

Histocompatibility (HLA) antigens

These inherited antigens, located on the sixth chromosome of the leukocytes, can be useful in the early diagnosis of ankylosing spondylitis and, to a lesser extent, the other seronegative spond-arthritic disorders (see Chapter 9). HLA-B27 is the marker of this group of conditions. Great caution must be taken in inter-

HLA-B27   preting a 'positive HLA' for the following reasons. HLA-B27 is present in 7% of normal people and in 50% of relatives of patients with ankylosing spondylitis (who will not necessarily get the disease). Therefore, the antigen is diagnostically useful only when a patient is thought to have reasonable clinical and radiological evidence of seronegative spondarthritis. It can also be helpful in undiagnosed cases of seronegative peripheral arthritis. Table 3.3 summarizes the most useful immunological tests.

Table 3.3   Basic immunology investigation profile

---
1. Tests for rheumatoid factor (RF)
2. ANA and DNA-binding
3. LE cells
4. Immunoelectrophoresis
5. WR and GCFT
6. ASO titre
7. HLA antigens

Blood chemistry

There are only a few chemical tests useful in the diagnosis of the more common rheumatic disorders: serum uric acid (in gout), calcium, phosphorus and alkaline phosphatase (in metabolic bone disease), acid phosphatase (in secondary prostatic cancer), and muscle enzymes (in myopathies and polymyositis).

Serum uric acid (SUA)

Hyper-
uricaemia

This should be requested in all cases of undiagnosed arthritis, as gout can masquerade as practically any acute arthritis. The blood urea and creatinine should also be requested because renal dysfunction leads to hyperuricaemia, as well as being a result of chronic gout (see Chapter 10). If the SUA is raised it should always be repeated. Hyperuricaemia may be secondary to polycythaemia, leukaemia and drug therapy (notably diuretics). The SUA is normally below 0.4 mmol/l and small amounts above this level are not usually very significant.

Serum calcium, phosphate and phosphatases

Osteomalacia

These are important in the diagnosis of osteomalacia (which can be a cause of backache, weakness and aching of the legs), and in the much less common condition hyperparathyroidism (which can underlie crystal deposition disease, osteoporosis and other bone lesions). A high alkaline phosphatase is also found in liver disease, but here abnormal liver function tests, including gamma GT are also found.

Serum acid and alkaline phosphatases

Prostate
carcinoma

These are raised in prostate carcinoma with bone secondaries and should be requested in males with backache and a raised ESR. It is the tartrate-stable acid phosphatase, which is raised above 6.2 IU/l in prostate cancer, and not the tartrate labile acid phosphatase, that matters.

Serum muscle enzymes (SME)

These may be raised in myopathies, muscular dystrophies and polymyositis. The creatinine phosphokinase (CPK) is the most commonly requested SME, values being normally less than 100 IU/l.

Plasma proteins and electrophoresis

Unlike immunoglobulins, these give information about albumin and fibrinogen as well as globulins. The alpha-2-globulin is an

Diagnosis and assessment

'acute phase reactant' which, when elevated, indicates tissue destruction in the early phases of rheumatic disease. A raised gammaglobulin indicates antibody formation and is more likely to be seen in the later states. A very high gammaglobulin level may occur in connective tissue diseases, in sarcoidosis and in myelomatosis where an abnormal band indicating a paraprotein is characteristic.

Urine tests

Proteinuria
A routine urine test (for protein, blood and sugar) should always be carried out. Proteinuria may be the first sign of a collagen disease such as polyarteritis, may represent Bence Jones protein in myeloma, or in rheumatoid disease may indicate urinary infection, nephropathy due to drugs (such as gold or penicillamine) or (much less commonly) secondary amyloid disease. If proteinuria persists a 24 hour urine specimen should be requested; more than 0.15 g protein/24 hours is abnormal, over 1 g/24 hours is found when there is renal tubular damage, and in nephrosis well over 5 g protein/24 hours can occur.

Blood in the urine

Haematuria
This is often found to be of no significance, but should be investigated if persistent. Haematuria is an early sign of polyarteritis. It is rarely seen when there is renal damage due to penicillamine (proteinuria is a much more common side-effect of this drug).

Midstream specimen (MSU)

A midstream specimen of urine (MSU) should be sent when routine analysis shows an abnormality or when urinary infection is suspected. A cell count should be carried out and the specimen may show red blood cells, casts or bacteria. When organisms are present antibiotic sensitivities are carried out.

The 24 hour calcium excretion in urine is decreased (below 2.5 mmol/24 hours) in osteomalacia and raised (above 7.5 mmol/24 hours) in hyperparathyroidism.

Synovial fluid analysis

It is possible for the general practitioner to examine synovial fluid after aspiration from a knee joint. The fluid is normally clear yellow and viscous – it forms a cohesive thread when dropped from a syringe. 'Inflammatory' fluids are turbid, green or yellowish and of low viscosity. A specimen of fresh fluid should be sent to the laboratory for the following tests.

Cells: a *cell count* (as well as morphology) should be requested, as some fluids in osteoarthritis contain up to 2000 cells/mm^3 whereas fluids from inflammatory arthritis are likely to contain ten times as many cells.

Crystals: urate crystals are diagnostic of gout, pyrophosphate crystals of chondrocalcinosis. A polarizing microscope is necessary to accurately identify these crystals.

Bacteria: found in septic arthritis (including tuberculous arthritis), the organisms are identified and their antibiotic sensitivities determined.

Chemistry: lysozomal enzymes, such as acid phosphatase and hydrolases, are raised in the synovial fluid of inflammatory arthritis. This can be useful when the cell count is not unduly raised – the acid phosphatase (total, not tartrate-stable) will be found to be at least twice as high as the serum acid phosphatase.

The interpretation of other characteristics of the synovial fluid (such as cell types, immunoglobulins and complement levels) can be difficult and are best left to the rheumatologist.

Early diagnosis: indications for referral for further opinion

When a patient presents for the first time with 'rheumatism' or 'arthritis' the general practitioner may or may not make a diagnosis. He may suspect a certain condition and this may be confirmed by appropriate investigation. If, however, the diagnosis still remains in doubt, treatment can only be non-specific or palliative and it would be wise to seek the opinion of a rheumatologist. There are other situations where this may be desirable. Where it is considered that treatment will eventually be surgical, an orthopaedic opinion should be sought, and the rheumatologist is in a better position to advise on the diagnosis and treatment of 'medical' cases; he has a wide background training in general (internal) medicine, is skilled in the use of local treatment (such as manipulation, splinting and steroid injections) and is usually adept in prescribing physiotherapy.

Need for referral

In general, the following may be given as indications for referral for specialist opinion:

(1) When there is doubt about the diagnosis.

When to refer

(2) When special investigations are required, or the interpretation of investigations previously ordered by the practi-

tioner is unclear. Certain procedures, such as the examination of synovial fluid using a polarizing microscope, biopsy and arthroscopy are best carried out by a rheumatologist.

(3) When treatment has been ineffective or only partly effective. Perhaps more than in any other specialty, the rheumatologist is as much concerned with treatment as with diagnosis! The assessment and treatment of arthritis is a highly complicated business requiring expertise, experience and understanding. Referral to the hospital also provides an opportunity for the patient to benefit from the skills of paramedical workers (particularly physiotherapists, occupational therapists, and medical social workers).

The referral letter   The referral letter should contain all basic information but should not be *too* long. It is important that this letter should include the following points:

(1) Previous rheumatic history, previous treatments and their effects.
(2) Relevant family history.
(3) Duration and brief history of the present complaint.
(4) Principal physical signs found by the practitioner.
(5) Results of any investigations.
(6) Previous drug therapy, effect and any allergies.
(7) Current drug therapy.
(8) Socio-economical matters: information about life at home, at work and recreations enjoyed.
(9) Brief information about general health, important previous illnesses and operations.
(10) Brief information about the psychological background.

Effect of the psyche on rheumatism

Assessment of the 'psychological overlay' – Psychological and emotional disturbances – 'Pure' psychogenic rheumatism

It will be observed that a whole chapter in this book has been devoted to psychological factors as they affect rheumatism and arthritis. This reflects their tremendous importance in modification of symptoms and the need to recognize their existence and their severity in relation to existing organic disease.

While 'pure' psychogenic rheumatism – that is, rheumatic pain entirely due to psychological disturbance – is uncommon though occasional cases do appear, the *modification* of organic rheumatic disease including arthritis by mental reactions is extremely common. Such psychological disturbances, often inaccurately called 'overlay', fall into three categories: anxiety reactions, depressive states and hysterical-conversion reactions (including malingering and compensation neurosis, often known as 'swinging the lead'). It is very important to assess the *degree* of psychological overlay in relation to the magnitude of the physical abnormalities, treatment and prognosis being greatly dependent on this.

Assessment of the 'psychological overlay'

Psychological overlay

Psychiatrists dislike the term 'psychological overlay' as this is never a satisfactory way of describing mental disorder. Nevertheless, it is a useful umbrella term to include all the various types of psychological abnormality in relation to their importance in a given case. The degree of 'psychological overlay' is often readily assessed by the experienced physician by observing certain features:

(1) The description of pain: florid description of pain or unusual distribution of referral ('all the way down one side of the body').
(2) Unusual accompanying symptoms: such as shaking of a limb or a feeling of 'swelling' of a part (there being no obvious visible swelling).
(3) Overreaction to examination: for example, back movements are unduly limited by obvious muscle spasm or extreme degrees of local tenderness on palpation.
(4) Undue aggravation or amelioration of pain by various factors: for example, complete disappearance of pain while away on holiday, its reappearance on return from holiday, worsening of symptoms in association with emotional factors (such as, stress, bereavement).
(5) Lack of sleep disturbance even though daytime pain is said to be severe.
(6) Complete lack of response to analgesics, even large doses of strong analgesics.

Psychological and emotional disturbances – their manifestations in rheumatology

After deciding that a significant degree of 'psychological overlay' is present, having assessed its degree in relation to the magnitude of the physical disorder, the next step is to try to recognize the category of mental upset, usually anxiety, depression, a combination of anxiety and depression or a hysterical conversion reaction.

Reactions

Anxiety

Anxiety reactions

Anxiety reactions are usually easily recognized. A common example is where the pain of cervical spondylosis is aggravated by marked spasm of the neck muscles. If the cause for anxiety cannot be readily removed, it can be alleviated by a tranquillizer drug such as diazepam.

48

Depression

Depressive reactions

Depression can vary from mild, reactive states to severe depressive illness (either unipolar or part of manic-depressive psychosis). The treatment of severe depression should be left to a psychiatrist, but complete or nearly complete response of pain to antidepressant drugs provides proof of a large depressive overlay. Some of these drugs (such as amitryptyline and Prothiaden) give relief of anxiety as well as depression. This is sometimes classified as agitated depression, as opposed to typical endogenous depression where there is retardation rather than agitation, imipramine usually being preferred to the tricyclic drugs. It is important to realize that patients with chronic rheumatoid arthritis often appear to become worse as a result of depression, with arthritis sometimes becoming deceptively 'active'. When this is suspected a trial of antidepressant drugs often results in an extraordinary degree of clinical improvement.

Hysterical-conversion reactions

Hysterical paralysis

Classical hysterical-conversion reactions such as hemi-anaesthesia, 'clavus' headache (piercing like a nail) or hysterical paralysis of one or more limb are less commonly seen, but mild conversion reactions in the form of malingering are of course common in practice. Here the salient feature is the presence of physical signs considerably out of proportion to the symptoms. This 'compensionitis' is nearly always present to some degree in patients attending for insurance examinations and legal reports relating to pain persisting after an injury at work or a road traffic accident. As a rule, complete resolution of a malingering problem must await settlement of the legal situation.

'Pure' psychogenic rheumatism

As mentioned above this is much less common but every now and then a true example turns up. Certain criteria should be satisfied in order to make this diagnosis:

Criteria for psychogenic rheumatism

(1) The symptoms are atypical or florid.
(2) Organic disease is excluded (or is judged to be minimal in relation to the psychological upset).
(3) There are clear-cut features of anxiety, depression or hysteria.

49

(4) There is a very adequate response to psychotropic drugs or other appropriate psychiatric treatment.

Purely psychogenic rheumatism is often rewarding to diagnose and treat. For example, backache associated with depressive illness may respond to a few weeks treatment with an antidepressant drug. Unless the psychogenic origin of the pain is recognized the patient may be subjected to weeks of completely useless and time-wasting physiotherapy, admission to hospital, or even surgery. Orthopaedic surgeons are aware of this and are often reluctant to operate whenever there is a strong psychological history, even where surgery would otherwise be indicated.

5 Basic management of arthritis and rheumatism

Pain relief – Disease activity and its reduction – Improvement of mobility and function – Analgesics – Anti-inflammatory drugs – Practical procedures – Physiotherapy – Occupational therapy and rehabilitation

Obviously the first aim in treatment of patients with rheumatism or arthritis is to relieve pain. We must then consider how to control joint swelling, how to alleviate stiffness, how to improve mobility and function, how to minimize deformity (and, where possible, abolish it).

Pain relief
Simple local measures

Though hardly ever recommended in hospital, a good rub with a liniment or ointment may be greatly appreciated. A paper collar covered with cloth helps to ease a stiff neck, a covered hot-water bottle or electric blanket is a simple way to relieve back pain, a soft pad inserted into the heel of the shoe eases the pain of
Heat and cold plantar fasciitis. Some patients find that cold applications (applied by covered icepacks or a cooling aerosol spray) are more effective than heat; only trial in the individual patient will decide this. In hospital physiotherapy departments heat or cold are always applied in order to give analgesia and muscle relaxation prior to exercise therapy.

51

Simple analgesic drugs

Purely pain relieving (as opposed to anti-inflammatory) drugs are discussed below (see p. 57).

Muscle relaxant drugs

It does not really matter whether the so-called muscle relaxants, such as diazepam and orphenadrine, really have a significant relaxing effect on voluntary muscle or whether they simply relieve anxiety, thereby relieving muscle spasm. However, they have an important synergistic action with analgesics and should always be considered, particularly when planning relief of pain due to acute musculoskeletal disorders such as disc lesions. When a patient with an acute lumbar disc lesion is admitted to hospital he is put on a combination of diazepam (or similar relaxant) with a weak analgesic such as paracetamol several times daily. Strong analgesics such as dihydrocodeine (DF118) are prescribed 'PRN' only. In patients treated at home by the general practitioner the lack of 'controlled environment' (complete rest, nursing, etc.) as in a hospital situation may compel the practitioner to resort to stronger analgesics on a more frequent and regular basis. The value of regular relaxant drugs should still not be overlooked. A drug combination as has been mentioned can be used, or alternatively a combined preparation such as Equagesic (which contains the mild analgesics ethoheptazine and aspirin and the anti-anxiety drug meprobamate). As mentioned in Chapter 4 underlying depression makes pain seem more severe and an antidepressive drug (such as amitriptyline (Tryptizol), imipramine or dothiepin (Prothiaden) is indicated, either alone or together with an anti-anxiety preparation.

Anti-inflammatory drugs

The non-steroidal anti-inflammatory drugs, occasionally systemic steroids, are indicated for rheumatic pain syndromes associated with inflammation – particularly inflammation of joints (arthritis). When inflammation subsides pain is relieved, so these drugs work indirectly.

Steroid injections

When pain arises from inflammation of one or a few joints, or from a specific area of inflamed connective tissue (such as teno-

Steroid
injections in
practice

synovitis), injection of steroid into the joint or in relation to inflamed connective tissue rapidly relieves pain. The question is often asked whether family doctors should give steroid injections. I have no doubt that they should familiarize themselves with the use of local steroids for soft tissue rheumatism. Regarding intra-articular injections, some practitioners choose to inject joints, others prefer to leave this to the specialist because of the technical difficulties which sometimes arise, and because of the fear of complications – septic arthritis being the most notorious. The selection of joints for injection is an art acquired by practice, and experience is particularly required to successfully inject the small joints of the fingers and toes.

Small joint
injections

Physiotherapy

Local applications of heat and cold have been mentioned. Other procedures, such as the application of short wave diathermy, ultrasound, cervical and lumbar traction, are best left to the skills of the physiotherapist.

Manipulation

Manipulation
in practice

Spinal
manipulation

Patients should be persuaded to realize that in order to have manipulative therapy it is not necessary to consult osteopaths or chiropractors. Many rheumatologists are good manipulators and most physiotherapists are trained in Maitland techniques (see page 71). It is a good idea for family doctors to become familiar with simple manipulative procedures. These are easily learned, though to become skilful (that is, gentle and efficient) experience is required. Spinal manipulation is not indicated in all cases of backache and it is important to get to know which conditions often respond to manipulation, such as acute intervertebral joint derangements, and which do not, such as slowly progressive, 'pulpy' lumbar disc prolapses. Other types of physiotherapy, such as lumbar traction and exercise therapy, can be useful in conjunction with manipulation of the spine.

Acupuncture

This, the most emotive subject of them all, will continue to be viewed with distrust and disbelief as long as medical traditionalists refuse to recognize that acupuncture as practised in the 'western' manner, leaving out the hocuspocus and mystique, can relieve pain and muscle spasm. This is not entirely placebo

treatment. Unfortunately, controlled trials are extremely difficult, so there is still no proof of its efficacy (see also page 69).

Disease activity and its reduction
Disease activity

Disease activity is an important concept in rheumatology in
relation to the current severity of the disease and its control.
Active and inactive arthritis Arthritis is said to be 'active' or 'inactive' (active refers to active
inflammation). Active joints are painful, often swollen, and may
contain excessive fluid. Inactive arthritis is like an extinct
volcano – the joint is not painful (there may be some discomfort
for mechanical reasons) though it may still be swollen or
deformed. The volcano may 'erupt' (become active) at any time.
This applies to the synovial joints of the spine, as in ankylosing
spondylitis and sacroiliitis as well as in peripheral arthritis.

General disease activity General disease activity applies to the sum total of inflammatory parameters at a given time. It can be assessed and com-
pared at intervals, as when judging the effect of an anti-inflammatory drug. Useful parameters in the assessment of disease
activity are:

(1) Degree of pain.
(2) Duration of morning stiffness.
(3) Degree of joint swelling.
(4) Weight loss.
(5) Deterioration in general health.
(6) Degree of fatigue and its time of onset.
(7) Degree of anaemia (which parallels disease activity).

A good idea of the disease activity in a case of rheumatoid
arthritis can be gained by bedside assessment using these
parameters. Serial assessments of activity guide the physician
in therapy – whether hospitalization is required, whether a
stronger anti-inflammatory agent is indicated.

A quantitative comparison of disease activities can be
arrived at by grading and summating the various parameters. In
the above list the parameters may be graded 0 (absent), 1
(slight), 2 (moderate) and 3 (severe). The maximum total will be 24
and the disease activity A can be expressed as a percentage of
the total possible activity:

$$A = \frac{\Sigma \text{ activities of parameters}}{24} \times 100$$

For example, in a moderately active case of rheumatoid arthritis the sum of activities of parameters could be 14 so $A = 14/24 \times 100 = 58\%$. This is *generalized* disease activity.

Local disease activity When one or only a few joints are considered, this is *local* disease activity. Resting an active joint and prescribing anti-inflammatory drugs may be effective, but often aspiration of the joint and an intra-articular steroid injection are required and occasionally persistent synovitis requires surgical synovectomy or the injection of radioactive isotopes. Reduction of generalized disease activity requires consideration of several possibilities:

Reducing generalized disease activity

(1) Resting active joints (splinting where required).
(2) Resting the body as a whole (by bedrest, in home or in hospital).
(3) Prescribing non-steroidal anti-inflammatory drugs.
(4) In persistently active cases of rheumatoid arthritis prescribing gold, penicillamine, systemic steroids or immunosuppressive drugs.
(5) Injecting corticosteroids into persistently active joints.
(6) Controlling intercurrent disease (such as, infections).
(7) Actively treating persistent anaemia.

The above have to be considered in all cases of active polyarthritis, whether seropositive or seronegative. The exception is ankylosing spondylitis; in patients with this condition spinal exercises rather than rest is desirable, particularly after pain is controlled by suitable anti-inflammatory drugs (see Chapter 9). Steroid injections are not given into spinal or sacroiliac joints (but may be useful for the peripheral arthritis which is occasionally seen in ankylosing spondylitis). Relatively small doses of anti-inflammatory drugs are needed and systemic steroids are hardly ever advocated.

Improvement of mobility and function

Lower limb arthritis Whenever arthritis of moderate or severe degree affects the lower limb there is some loss of mobility. Inability to get around properly is a severe handicap. The life of an arthritic patient is transformed by improvement in his mobility, as is so often evident after a successful total hip replacement when pain is relieved and mobility regained.

Upper limb arthritis

Arthritis affecting the upper limb more or less restricts the patient's daily activities (ADL) including dressing, washing, eating, writing and his work in general. While hand surgery is often successful we still have a long way to go before operations on the upper limb achieve the level of hip surgery. Meanwhile, the occupational therapist can be very helpful in this respect (see below).

What can be done to improve mobility and function? The following can be considered:

(1) Physiotherapy (mainly exercise therapy).
(2) Occupational therapy (activities and, where appropriate, the provision of self-help devices).
(3) Appliances (special footware, arch supports, collars and lumbar supports).
(4) Crutches and walking sticks.
(5) Wheelchairs.
(6) Surgery for the joints.

Surgery to improve mobility and function

Surgery to improve mobility and function lies in one of the following three categories of operation for joints severely damaged by arthritis.

Arthrodesis

This converts a painful, unstable joint into a stiff, stable pain-free one. The following are often arthrodesed: the wrist, the first carpometacarpal joint at the base of the thumb, the ankle and the knee.

Osteotomy

This (a) corrects a fixed deformity, such as genu valgum, and (b) relieves pain – partially by correcting mechanical disadvantage but also in a non-specific manner.

Arthroplasty

This includes (a) removal of the joint (pseudarthrosis) such as in Fowler's or Helals' operation where the metatarsal heads are excised, (b) replacement arthroplasty (joint replacement) where one or both joint surfaces are replaced by a prosthesis, the classical example being total hip replacement.

Analgesics

Analgesics are pain-relieving drugs and they do not usually have anti-inflammatory activity. Though anti-inflammatory drugs are much more important than analgesics in the management of inflammatory rheumatic disorders such as rheumatoid arthritis, analgesics are nearly always required as well, and they are of course important in patients with osteoarthritis, backache and soft tissue rheumatism.

The analgesics used in rheumatology may be classified as follows:

(1) Weak analgesics for routine use (such as paracetamol and aspirin).
(2) Rather stronger analgesics for occasional use (such as codeine and dextropropoxyphene).
(3) Moderately powerful analgesics for occasional use (such as dihydrocodeine and pentazocine).
(4) Very powerful analgesics for only very occasional use such as pethidine and dipipanone).

It will be noted that morphine and heroin do not appear on this list. These addictive drugs should never be used for relieving pain in musculoskeletal disorders. In, for example, an acute lumbar disc lesion it is good policy to put the patient to rest and prescribe something like codeine co. together with diazepam or a similar agent at regular intervals. In the domiciliary situation some practitioners will not be able to resist an intramuscular injection of pethidine, but this should not be repeated several times.

Weak analgesics
Paracetamol (Panadol)

This can be taken freely at 3–4 hour intervals without fear of side-effects. The preparation Lobak conveniently combines paracetamol with a tranquillizer, chlormezanone, and is useful when some sedation is required. Paracetamol should be avoided in liver disease and very large doses can produce severe liver damage.

Aspirin

This is anti-inflammatory in large doses (12 tablets = 3.6 g/day) but only analgesic in small doses (up to 6–8 tablets daily). It can cause dyspepsia, less likely with soluble aspirin or enteric-coated aspirin preparations. Some patients are hypersensitive to aspirin and develop skin rashes or asthma and some tend to get 8th nerve toxicity with relatively small doses – this is especially likely in elderly patients and those with chronic ear disease. Small doses of aspirin produce hyperuricaemia, so should not be used in gout.

Diflunisal (Dolobid)

This analogue of aspirin has a prolonged action lasting several hours. Some patients find that one tablet twice daily is a good analgesic, but despite claims to the contrary there is little or no anti-inflammatory effect at this dosage.

Stronger analgesics

These are for occasional use, perhaps supplementing regular aspirin or paracetamol medication.

Codeine

This can be given in tab. codeine co. which contains aspirin as well, or by itself as codeine phosphate. Soluble codeine (Codis) tablets contain 500 mg soluble aspirin with 8 mg codeine phosphate. Taken regularly codeine tends to constipate, and can therefore be a useful analgesic for the arthritis associated with ulcerative colitis and Crohn's disease.

Dextropropoxyphene

This is usually prescribed as Distalgesic which contains this drug together with paracetamol. It is now becoming clear that there is probably a mild addictive effect, so patients tend to 'like it' and believe (wrongly) that it is a strong analgesic. For this reason it is unwise to prescribe dextropropoxyphene routinely, and particular care should be taken in giving it with central nervous system depressants.

Moderately powerful analgesics

These are only for occasional use.

Dihydrocodeine (DF 118)

This is rather stronger than codeine, and causes a similar degree of constipation. One or two 30 mg tablets of dihydrocodeine tartrate are given 6 hourly as required, preferably not regularly. Unlike pentazocine this is well tolerated by ambulant patients.

Pentazocine (Fortral)

This is useful in recumbent patients (such as those on bedrest for disc lesions) but tends to cause central nervous system toxicity in ambulant patients. It is more potent when given by intramuscular injection, 30–60 mg every few hours (but carefully, as high doses may produce respiratory depression, reversed by naloxone).

Very powerful analgesics

These are potentially addictive, so should only be used very occasionally with great care.

Pethidine and dipipanone

The former is given in 50 mg tablets or as a very occasional intramuscular injection. Dipipanone (Diconal) is given in 10 mg tablets, and also include cyclizine (an antihistamine) to prevent nausea – this is a respiratory depressant and should be avoided in elderly patients and those with incipient cardiorespiratory disease.

Anti-inflammatory drugs

In rheumatology anti-inflammatory drugs are classified as (a) non-steroidal anti-inflammatory drugs, a large variety of preparations being available, (b) systemic steroids, which are very strong anti-inflammatory agents and only indicated in certain situations, and (c) specific drugs for the treatment of rheumatoid arthritis (principally gold and penicillamine), and (d) immunosuppressive and immunostimulant drugs.

Non-steroidal anti-inflammatory drugs (NSAIDs)

These are used especially in the inflammatory arthropathies, systemic connective tissue diseases, ankylosing spondylitis and

Uses of NSAID gout. They are not really of much help in soft tissue rheumatism and are only of limited value in backache and osteoarthritis. They have different effects (and side-effects) in different people. It is, therefore, often necessary to 'ring the changes' of the NSAID, but at the same time it is wise to know and understand the use of a limited number of them. One could first try the effect of indomethacin which is a time-proven powerful anti-inflammatory drug and when used properly (as described below) is usually well tolerated. Should it be ineffective or not well tolerated, another NSAID such as Naprosyn could be substituted, or else one of the newer preparations such as Methrazone or Feldene.

Aspirin

In full dosage (10–12 tablets, or 3–3.6 g/day) aspirin is anti-inflammatory as well as analgesic. Many rheumatologists still use it as the first drug of choice in rheumatoid arthritis. Family doctors are wary that their patients on continued aspirin therapy
Dyspepsia or may develop dyspepsia due to gastric irritation and sometimes
haematemesis haematemesis due to acute ulceration of the mucosa. This is made less likely if aspirin is prescribed in the enteric-coated form (Enseal aspirin), as aloxiprin (Palaprin forte), or as benorylate (Benoral, a paracetamol ester of acetylsalicylic acid). It should be noted that when benorylate 10 ml b.d. is prescribed the patient is having a nearly maximum dose of salicylate, so should be careful about taking any extra aspirins

Table 5.1 Alphabetical list of NSAIDs

Alclofenac (Prinalgin)
Azaproprazone (Rheumox)
Benoxaprofen (Opren)
Diclofenac (Voltarol)
Fenclofenac (Flenac)
Fenoprofen (Fenopron)
Feprazone (Methrazone)
Flufenamic acid (Meralen)
Flurbiprofen (Froben)
Ibuprofen (Brufen)
Indomethacin (Indocid)
Ketoprofen (Alrheumat, Orudis)
Mefanemic acid (Ponstan)
Naproxen (Naprosyn)
Phenylbutazone (Butazolidin) and oxyphenbutazone (Tanderil)
Piroxicam (Feldene)
Sulindac (Clinoril)
Tolmetin (Tolectin)

(such as to relieve headache) – 8th nerve toxicity (deafness and tinnitus) is a particularly common side-effect in elderly patients.

Table 5.1 shows alphabetically, NSAIDs (other than aspirin preparations). The trade name of the drug is given in brackets after the official name.

NSAIDs and their actions

Alclofenac
Alclofenac can be quickly dismissed because, although its anti-inflammatory effect is considerable (and there is some evidence of a delayed, specific effect), frequent severe skin rashes obviate its routine use.

Azapropazone
Azapropazone chemically resembles phenylbutazone but its actions resemble those of proprionic acid derivatives. In my experience it is quite effective in some patients and is not often toxic. Although not often advocated in gout, it could be useful here as it has a marked uricosuric as well as anti-inflammatory effect. Gastric intolerance is quite common. Like many other NSAIDs it potentiates anticoagulants so should not be used in patients having these. The *average dose* is 300 mg q.i.d.

Benoxaprofen
Benoxaprofen is a new drug with some delay in effect. Severe photosensitive skin rashes are unfortunately not uncommon.

Diclofenac
Diclofenac is an amino-phenylacetic acid. It does not interfere with anticoagulants, but concurrent aspirin administration lowers the blood levels. It is said to be equipotent with indomethacin and is certainly worth a trial when the latter is ineffective or toxic. Side-effects of diclofenac are mainly gastrointestinal and occur at an early stage. *Average dose* is 25 mg t.i.d.

Fenclofenac
Fenclofenac is a new drug, still in the clinical trial stage at the time of writing. The *average dose* is 300 mg b.d.

Fenoprofen
Fenoprofen is one of the proprionic acids, and has been shown to be more potent than ketoprofen and ibuprofen though more likely to cause gastrointestinal side-effects. It also has a rather unusually marked immediate analgesic effect. *Starting average dose* is 300 or 600 mg q.i.d.

Feprazone
Feprazone is another new drug which I think has great promise and may turn out to be a real rival to indomethacin. *Average dose* is 200 mg t.i.d. after food.

Flufenamic acid
Flufenamic acid appeared some time ago when, for some reason, it lost popularity and has now reappeared under the proprietary name of Meralen. Like mefanemic acid it is a fenamate, the *average dose* being 200 mg t.i.d. with food. It is

61

claimed that it both inhibits prostaglandin synthesis and antagonizes its action. It may potentiate anticoagulants, also sulphonylurea hypoglycaemic drugs, so care should be taken in diabetics taking these.

Flurbiprofen and ibuprofren

Flurbiprofen is a 'cousin' of ibuprofren, a phenylalkanoic acid. It is more potent than ibuprofren, but not perhaps in the larger doses now advocated. The *average dose* of flurbiprofen is 50 mg or 100 mg t.i.d. Unlike ibuprofen it is a potent inhibitor of platelet aggregation and one of the most potent inhibitors of prostaglandin synthesis. It does not interfere with anticoagulant therapy, but can irritate the stomach and is contraindicated if there is a history of peptic ulcer.

Ibuprofen, a proprionic acid derivative, was originally advocated in a dose of 200 mg t.i.d. when it is only weakly anti-inflammatory. This proved overcautious and there is improved activity in a *dose of 400 mg t.i.d.* or q.i.d. It has some analgesic properties and is often a 'first drug' in family practice, though rheumatologists would not consider it an anti-inflammatory drug of choice in rheumatoid arthritis. It has the great advantage of few side-effects but, although not usually irritant to the gastric mucosa, this is not always the case and should be only used very carefully in cases of peptic ulcer.

Indomethacin

Indomethacin is the 'classic', potent anti-inflammatory drug preferred by many rheumatologists for the treatment of arthritis, gout and ankylosing spondylitis. Immediate side-effects, particularly neurological (headaches, dizziness), can usually be obviated by starting indomethacin as a single 50 mg capsule taken with fluids (preferably milk) last thing before retiring. A more prolonged effect following a single nightly dose can be obtained by prescribing the long-acting preparation, Indocid R 75 mg. A single dose of 50 or 75 mg at night is often sufficient, but if necessary a supplementary dose of 25 mg can be given next morning. Should it cause dyspepsia, indomethacin may be prescribed as suppositories (100 mg at night). Patients on long-term indomethacin therapy should watch carefully for dyspepsia, as large ulcers on the greater curvature can develop, although these usually heal when the drug is stopped. When given at night indomethacin is often said to help sleep (though perhaps this is simply due to relief of pain) and it has a pronounced effect in relieving morning stiffness the next day. The drug is not advised for elderly patients who do not tolerate it well (naproxen is a useful alternative here). It is antipyretic and may mask the symptoms of infection, so it should be used with extra care; it does not potentiate anticoagulants. It is unwise to prescribe indomethacin for very long periods in patients with osteoarthritis of weight bearing joints – there is some evidence that it can lead to bone destruction in osteoarthritis of the hip and produce a form of avascular necrosis which surgeons call 'indomethacin arthropathy'.

Ketoprofen

Ketoprofen is a proprionic acid derivative about equipotent to ibuprofen and aspirin. *Average dose* is 50 mg t.i.d. with food. Like ibuprofen, its great advantage is lack of side-effects – it is a very safe drug for use in general practice – but, although theoretically it should be a fairly powerful NSAID, it is only occasionally useful in rheumatoid arthritis as an alternative to aspirin when this is not well tolerated.

Mefanemic acid

Mefanemic acid is a fenamate, its activity and toxicity being similar to flufenamine acid. Its *average dose* is 500 mg t.i.d. Unlike flufenamic acid it can be safely given to children (as a paediatric suspension, 50 mg per 5 ml).

Naproxen

Naproxen, probably the most effective proprionic acid derivative, is almost as potent as indomethacin and has become a popular alternative, being effective in about 60% of patients with rheumatoid arthritis (possibly in a certain subgroup of patients) and thus more effective than ibuprofen or ketoprofen for routine hospital use. It is also frequently used in general practice. The best dose, formerly quoted as 250 mg b.i.d., is now thought to be (*average dose*) 250 mg t.i.d. A dose of 500 mg may be given at night (as with indomethacin) to relieve early-morning stiffness. It does not potentiate oral coumarin anticoagulants and, apart from occasional nausea and indigestion, it is quite free from side-effects.

Phenyl-butazone

Phenylbutazone, a pyrazole, is of course the 'old man' of anti-inflammatory drugs and still the first choice of many rheumatologists in the treatment of acute gout and ankylosing spondylitis (see Chapters 10 and 9). However, it has largely been superseded by indomethacin and the newer NSAIDs because of the slight risk of haemotoxicity when given over a long period. Usually a safe *average dose* is 100 mg twice or three times daily; it is still wise to check regular monthly blood counts. Phenylbutazone has a relatively long half-life and its maximum effect may not be achieved for 1–3 weeks. Besides the danger of

BTZ toxicity

agranulocytosis, the potential side-effects are numerous:

Side-effects

dyspepsia and occasional peptic ulceration (less frequent with the coated variety, Butacote, or with oxyphenbutazone), various rashes, antithyroid activity (if prescribed for a patient with rheumatism or myopathy associated with hypothyroidism the symptoms often become worse), oedema due to water and salt retention (it should be avoided in cardiorenal disease), potentiation of tolbutamide and chlorpropamide in diabetics. Small doses of phenylbutazone are often given to elderly osteo-arthritic patients who often say it is their favourite drug. However, it must be remembered that over 25 patients die from haemorrhage due to aplastic anaemia every year and regular blood counts do not ensure against this as the haematological changes may occur extremely suddenly.

Piroxicam, sulindac and tolmetin Piroxicam is a recent drug which has a long half-life so can be given once daily (20 mg). Sulindac is an indene deriv-ative of indomethacin but is certainly less effective and probably not less toxic though headaches do not occur. The *average dose* is 200 mg b.i.d. Tolmetin also resembles Indocid chemically, but its action is more like the proprionic acid com-pounds; in other words it is mainly analgesic with only a minor anti-inflammatory effect. The *average dose* is 400 mg t.i.d.

Systemic corticosteroids

These are used in systemic connective-tissue disorders and in certain severe cases of rheumatoid arthritis. In rheumatology practice, the most frequent indication for steroids is *polymyalgia rheumatica*. This diagnosis is often made by family doctors, and before prescribing steroids it is wise to exclude possible underlying conditions, such as rheumatoid arthritis presenting with painful shoulders, malignant tumours, myeloma and subacute bacterial endocarditis (see Chapter 00). Systemic steroids are *not* normally indicated in osteoarthritis, gout, ankylosing spondylitis, back pain syndromes or soft-tissue rheumatism.

Small doses the rule Small doses of steroids is the rule in rheumatology, a total dose of 7.5 mg prednisolone rarely being exceeded except in certain connective-tissue diseases and sometimes polymyalgia. It is not good practice to give 'crash courses' of steroids, starting

Prescribing steroids with large doses and then reducing it in steps. The lowest pos-sible effective dose is found by prescribing prednisolone as 1 mg tablets and reducing the daily dose very slowly, perhaps by 1 mg per month. There is no need to consider other corticosteroid derivatives, as they are no better than prednisolone and often more toxic. Should steroids cause dyspepsia enteric coated tablets (2.5 mg) or soluble prednisolone phosphate dissolved in water can be given. There is no reason to prescribe ACTH (corticotrophin) in place of systemic steroids in general practice.

Side-effects and precautions in steroid use

The side-effects of steroids are well known and include the following:

Side-effects
of steroids

(1) 'Moon-face' and flushing.
(2) Oedema (hypertension due to sodium retention is not common with low doses).
(3) Spinal osteoporosis, leading to crush fractures of vertebrae.
(4) Peptic ulceration.
(5) Growth suppression in children.
(6) Dissemination of infection (facilitation of growth and spread of viruses and bacteria).
(7) Thinning of the skin and 'steroid bruising'.
(8) Impairment of glucose tolerance, precipitation of diabetes if latent, loss of blood sugar control in treated diabetics.
(9) Steroid cataracts, glaucoma.
(10) Steroid withdrawal syndrome (adrenal insufficiency following withdrawal).
(11) Psychiatric changes (insomnia, depression etc.).
(12) Aseptic necrosis of bone (steroid osteoarthropathy).
(13) Steroid myopathy.

Steroid
precautions

The following precautions should be observed in all patients on steroids:

(1) The patient must carry a 'steroid card' giving his address, doctor and current dose of steroid. (A 'steroid bracelet' is also a good idea, see Figure 5.1).
(2) The serum electrolytes should be reviewed in oedematous patients, especially those given diuretics.
(3) Calcium supplements or calcium/bone salts should be given to elderly patients.
(4) The chest should be X-rayed to exclude tuberculosis.
(5) The steroid dosage must be raised temporarily during stress, illness, operations or anaesthesia.
(6) Steroids must not be withdrawn suddenly.

Specific drugs in rheumatoid arthritis

These are principally gold, penicillamine and antimalarials; they are discussed further in Chapter 8.

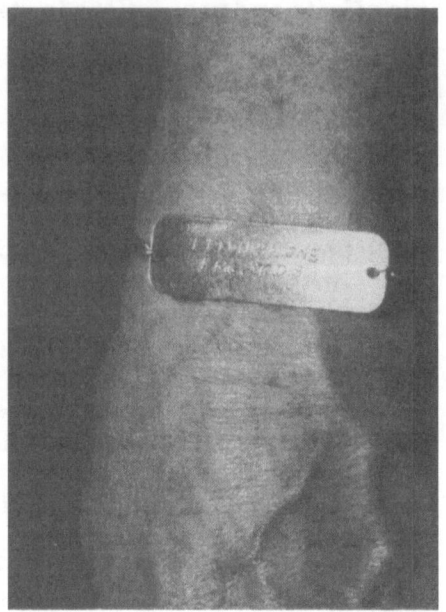

'Steroid bracelet' showing current prednisolone dosage

Figure 5.1

Immunosuppressive drugs

These drugs, which include cyclophosphamide and azathioprine, are sometimes used in difficult cases of rheumatoid arthritis, systemic connective-tissue disorders and neoplastic conditions such as myelomatosis which can present with rheumatic syndromes.

Azathioprine

The average dose of azathioprine is 50 mg b.i.d. Sometimes cyclizine hydrochloride is given initially to counteract nausea. The aim is to reduce the white cell count to 2000–3000/mm^3 and maintain it at this level. A complete blood count and platelet count is requested monthly and the blood should continue to be monitored.

Cyclo-
phosphamide

Cyclophosphamide is given as 50 mg t.i.d. or q.i.d. Side-effects, including loss of hair, can often be obviated by giving short, more intensive courses, for example during the first week of every month. Besides excessive neutropenia (the blood count must be monitored as above), other occasional side-effects of cyclophosphamide are haemorrhagic cystitis and sterility, so it should not be given to young patients.

Chlorambucil

Chlorambucil 5–7.5 mg/day may be added to another immunosuppressive drug, rather than being prescribed alone.

66

Immunostimulant drugs

Laevamisole The principal immunostimulant drug is laevamisole, occasionally used in refractory cases of rheumatoid arthritis. It is still under investigation.

Practical procedures in family practice

Practitioners should be familiar with the following techniques:

(1) Aspiration of effusions from some joints, especially the knee.
(2) Corticosteroid injections into soft tissues and into some joints.
(3) Basic manipulation of the spine.

Aspiration of joint effusions

There are two reasons for aspirating a large effusion: (a) to allow inspection and examination of the synovial fluid (see page 43), (b) to relieve pain or discomfort due to the effusion. It is also advisable to remove synovial fluid prior to injecting steroids, as the fluid both dilates and disintegrates the steroid, making it less efficacious. While aspiration of the knee joint is simple, the other joints are best avoided by the practitioner inexperienced in this technique. There is no need for preliminary local anaesthesia. In knee aspirations a no 21 needle attached to a 20 ml syringe is inserted just below the patella on the medial side with the knee fully extended. The plunger of the syringe is withdrawn; if fluid does not appear, the needle is withdrawn slightly and the procedure repeated.

Technique of
aspiration

Corticosteroid injections

Most rheumatologists would be lost should they be unable to give steroid injections when treating both inflammatory arthritis and soft tissue lesions. The practitioner should therefore familiarize himself with some basic injection techniques. Details are given in the author's *Concise Management of the Rheumatic Disorders* (Golding, 1979). The following are some useful practical points:

Steroid
injections

(1) Always aspirate effusions, if present, before injection of the steroid.

(2) When injecting small joints and soft tissues, mix the steroid with an equal volume of 2% lignocaine or similar local anaesthetic.

(3) Never inject the steroid where there is skin sepsis.

(4) Do not inject weight-bearing joints often.

(5) In tenosynovitis, inject into tendon sheath; avoid injection actually into tendons.

(6) Always warn patient about possible post-injection pain.

Manipulation of the spine

Basic techniques of mobilization of spinal joints by simple manipulation procedures should be understood by every general practitioner. There is nothing 'mysterious' about manipulation, which can be quickly learned by observing procedures (or attending a practical course), but knowing exactly when to manipulate under certain circumstances and perfecting the technique is a matter of experience. There are various types of spinal manipulation. Generally speaking, manipulation is particularly suitable for patients with the following conditions:

Indications for manipulation

(1) Acute backache (or neck pain) due to intervertebral joint derangements.

(2) Resolving acute disc lesions.

(3) Persisting back pain in young patients where one segment of the spine is found to be stiff.

(4) Some cases of chronic lumbago in older patients.

(5) Some cases of chronic sciatica (manipulation under anaesthesia is perhaps more suitable for these patients).

It is useless (and probably unwise) to try manipulating an acute prolapsed disc lesion where there is severe sciatica, the back movements are limited, straight-leg raising is greatly reduced on one or both sides, and a reflex is lost in one of the legs. Manipulation is of course contraindicated where there is an organic lesion of the vertebra (such as a tumour) or a cauda equina syndrome (shown by leg weakness, bladder and bowel dysfunction and 'saddle analgesia') where prompt surgical treatment is often required.

Contra-indications to manipulation

A simple rotational manipulation of the lumbar spine is carried out as follows. The patient lies on a couch with the pelvis rotated, the thigh hanging over the edge of the couch. The physician places one hand on the shoulder, the other on the hip, then suddenly pushing on the thigh rotates the thorax and pelvis in opposite directions.

Technique of manipulation

Acupuncture

Acupuncture is a new type of treatment in the western world. The role of stimulation of skin, subcutaneous tissue and periosteum by fine needles inserted at certain points has yet to be evaluated. It certainly does seem to be helpful in *some* patients with mild backache and neckache, particularly where there is referred pain and when muscle spasm is prominent.

Possible
theories of
acupuncture
If acupuncture does work, how? We are a long way from knowing this. One idea, based on the gate theory, is that the large (A-delta) pain fibres in the skin and subcutaneous tissues are stimulated by the acupuncture needle, thus cutting off the 'unpleasant' pain impulses conducted by the small unmyelinated C fibres at the 'gate' in the posterior horn and substantia gelatinosa of the spinal cord. In classical acupuncture there are hundreds of 'points' along the so-called 'meridians', but it is now usually believed that it is best to stimulate 'trigger points' which are tender and perhaps represent areas of muscle spasm. In acupuncture when there is pain relief it is often immediate, though effects delayed for a day or more are not uncommon. Soreness is often felt at the site of the needle punctures, but this soon disappears. Exacerbation of symptoms for a day or so afterwards occurs in some patients, especially those known as 'strong reactors'.

Basic
techniques of
acupuncture
Like manipulation, basic acupuncture techniques can be quite easily learned by attending courses run by physicians experienced in the art – there is no need to commit to memory the fourteen meridians and the myriad points and, like manipulation, skill in acupuncture appears to be associated with the acquisition of knowledge of when and where to try it, and how far to take it, rather than actual techniques. At the time of writing, only a handful of rheumatologists use acupuncture, which is rather odd, as I consider it a most useful method of relieving pain, especially referred pain, in the ubiquitous minor musculoskeletal conditions.

Physiotherapy

Physiotherapy is not taught to medical students as a part of the normal curriculum. The great majority of doctors, while knowing little or nothing about it, realize how useful it can be and most rheumatologists are conversant with its applications, its limitations and its possible prescription.

Importance of
physiotherapy

The least important use of physiotherapy is the soothing of pain by heat treatment. Its important use relates to the improvement of mobility and function which is essentially exercise therapy and mobilization of stiff joints. Therefore, we can happily dispense with the various forms of heat therapy (short wave diathermy, radiant heat, microwave) except for its use in muscle relaxation prior to exercise therapy.

The general practitioner may have access to an 'open' physiotherapy department in a nearby hospital and sometimes physiotherapists are available to attend patients at home. Otherwise physiotherapy is requested by communicating with an appropriate consultant, often a rheumatologist who has overall charge of the physiotherapy department. Sensible understanding of physiotherapy prescription is most important in the care of patients with rheumatism and arthritis.

Prescribing physiotherapy

Whenever physiotherapy is prescribed the following information should be supplied:

(1) The diagnosis.
(2) Other disorders which may have a bearing on the condition of the patient (such as heart failure, epilepsy, diabetes).
(3) Other current therapy (such as drugs, concomitant occupational therapy).
(4) The aim of treatment (such as mobilization of a stiff shoulder).
(5) The approximate duration of treatment (or number of treatments). In acute conditions daily treatment is often desirable, otherwise three sessions weekly for 2 or 3 weeks is usually sufficient.

(Note that details of the type of treatment are not mentioned in the above list: techniques should be left to the physiotherapist's judgement. While sometimes special techniques such as traction are advocated, the treatment can be varied at the discretion of the physiotherapist. I have no objection to this philosophy, but when I am specifically asked whether my directions can be altered, I reply 'yes', provided the patient is no worse as a result!)

Physiotherapy techniques

Details of various types of physiotherapy and their applications in rheumatology are described in my textbook (Golding, 1979). Commonly used techniques are:

(1) Heat/cold therapy.
(2) Exercise therapy.
(3) Hydrotherapy (exercises in the deep pool).
(4) Manipulation (physiotherapists normally use Maitland techniques).
(5) Ultrasound therapy (mainly for acute traumatic lesions).
(6) Electrical stimulation of muscles (mainly faradic stimulation of weak or wasted muscles (see Figure 5.2).
(7) Intermittent spinal traction (for cervical or lumbar disorders, see Chapter 11).

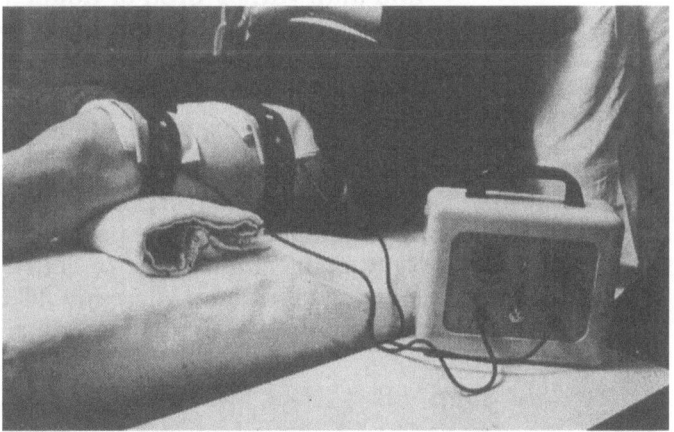

Figure 5.2

Faradic stimulation of quadriceps muscle in osteoarthritis of the knee

Hydrotherapy

This is very useful when there is general stiffness or several joints are affected, for exercising weight-bearing joints (such as the hip) and for helping achieve spinal mobility where this is greatly restricted, as in ankylosing spondylitis.

Home exercises

The physiotherapist often gives the patient exercises to do as 'homework', thereby bridging the gap between physiotherapy sessions which should be regarded as the 'tuition'. Exercises can also be advantageously prescribed by the practitioner, who should know a few simple exercises, for example extension exercises for backache: 'I'm going to teach you four exercises: two lying on the back (straight-leg raising and extending the back with the knees bent) and two lying on the stomach (straight-leg raising and arching the back with hands clasped behind)'. Exercises at home are very useful but all patients should be warned about certain aspects by teaching them the 'four golden rules':

Rules for exercise therapy

Rule I: Do not exercise during acute, very painful stages of the condition.

Rule II: No exercise should hurt more than a little – stop or postpone those that do.

Rule III: Exercise within a comfortable range of movement and until rather tired or aching, but not longer.

Rule IV: Exercise gently and often, rather than vigorously and occasionally.

Occupational therapy and rehabilitation

Doctors know even less about occupational therapy than physiotherapy. Yet both are an integral part of rehabilitation medicine, essential in the management of the patient with severe arthritis.

The practitioner should try to learn something of the indications for occupational therapy (OT) and liaise with hospital therapists who also visit patients' homes and supply

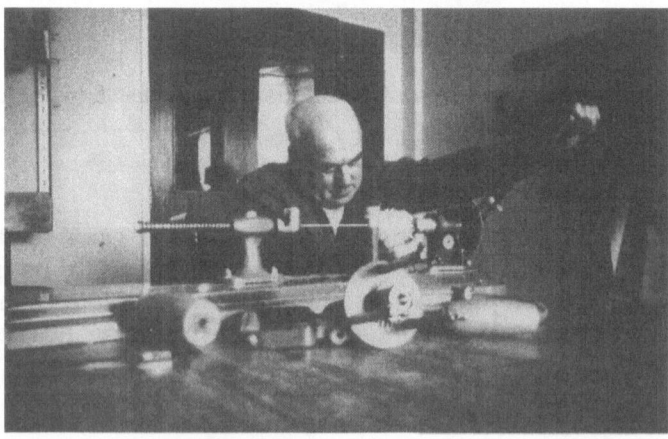

Brush-making machine to improve the range of shoulder movement

Figure 5.3

aids and implements where indicated. Just as physiotherapy does not mean merely soothing applications of heat, occupational therapy does not simply involve keeping the patient occupied, but uses specific activities aimed towards the improvement of mobility and function of joints (see for example, Figure 5.3).

Assessment

Before treatment is commenced, a full assessment is carried out by the occupational therapist, who records her findings for comparison before and after treatment. Such an assessment of a patient with chronic arthritis is shown in Table 5.2.

Table 5.2 Assessment of patient with chronic arthritis

1.	Medical assessment	the state of the arthritis and also disorders of other systems
2.	Functional assessment	the range of movement of the joints, deformities, muscle weakness and assessment of activities of daily living (ADL)
3.	Personality and mental assessment	
4.	Work assessment	
5.	Transportation	public transport and the ability to use a private car
6.	The home environment	initially the assessment of ADL at home is carried out in hospital occupational therapy departments with special units (such as kitchen, bedroom and bathroom); home visiting and the application of assessments to specific problems of the patient's home then follows.

Activities in the occupational therapy department

There are many types of activity to improve function. Examples are the use of clay in modelling, looms, woodwork and metalwork. Various games have an important role in physical and psychological rehabilitation.

Self-help devices

These aids are supplied only when function is sufficiently poor to impede performance of certain activities of daily living. For example, long-handled utensils compensate for poor elbow flexion, thick handles for incomplete grip. In the bathroom, the provision of hand-rails on the walls, and raising the toilet seat are helpful. An assortment of aids is usually kept in the occupational therapy department and many can be supplied by local authority occupational therapists.

SECTION 2
The Common Rheumatic Disorders

Soft-tissue (non-articular) rheumatism

Classification – Clinical varieties and treatment

Arthritis is the name given to diseases of joints and their attached structures. Rheumatic pain arising in tissues other than the joints is called *soft tissue or non-articular rheumatism.* At the same time it should be remembered that inflammation of a tendon (tenosynovitis) well away from a joint may be the first sign of rheumatoid arthritis, that is, arthritis may start with non-articular symptoms. Pain apparently arising in the soft tissues may in fact be referred from elsewhere (usually the spine). Generalized soft-tissue rheumatism (occurring in many areas at once) is a well-known feature of certain systemic illnesses. Non-articular rheumatism may also be a manifestation of certain psychological disturbances.

Classification

Soft-tissue rheumatism can be classified as follows:

(1) Local soft-tissue rheumatism affecting
    The fascia (fasciitis)
    The fat (panniculitis)
    The fibrous tissue (fibrositis)
    The muscles (myositis)
    The tendon sheaths (tenosynovitis)
    The bursae (bursitis)
    The tenoperiosteal junction (enthesopathy)

> The tissues surrounding joints (periarthritis or capsulitis)
>
> The ligaments (ligamentous strain or sprain)
>
> The peripheral nerves (entrapment neuropathy)

(2) Soft-tissue rheumatism referred from the spine or elsewhere

(3) Generalized rheumatism, occurring in
  Infectious diseases (such as influenza)
  Systemic connective tissue diseases (such as systemic lupus erythematosus – SLE)
  Endocrine disorders (such as hypothyroidism)
  Metabolic disorders (such as osteomalacia)
  Neurological disorders (such as polyneuritis)

(4) Psychogenic soft-tissue rheumatism
  Muscle spasm, fibrositis, certain painful neck and back syndromes, coccygodynia and xiphisternal pain are well-known examples of conditions which are wholly or largely dependent on abnormal psychological influences.

Clinical varieties and their treatment
Fasciitis

Plantar fasciitis

The best example is plantar fasciitis which causes pain in the heel spreading forward along the sole of the foot. Should fasciitis be bilateral (and especially if accompanied by Achilles tendinitis) the possibility that it might be *secondary* to some underlying arthritis should be considered. This could be rheumatoid arthritis, gout, or – most likely – a seronegative HLA-B27 positive arthropathy (see Chapter 9), such as ankylosing spondylitis or Reiter's disease. The common primary (idiopathic) plantar fasciitis is often associated with a little calcaneal 'spur' seen in the X-ray (see Figure 6.1) which is a consequence of chronic inflammation (a periosteal reaction) and the spur itself does not influence the symptoms (unless it is very large indeed). Sometimes a fuzzy, eroded 'spur' is seen in secondary plantar fasciitis.

Spurs on X-ray

Treatment of plantar fasciitis

The pain is due to an enthesopathy, inflammation of the plantar fascia where it joins the heel bone, so this is the point to infiltrate with a mixture of local anaesthetic, steroid (such as triamcinolone acetonide) and hyaluronidase (a spreading agent). Plantar fasciitis is often a result of chronic stretching of the fascia on account of pes planus, when arch supports will

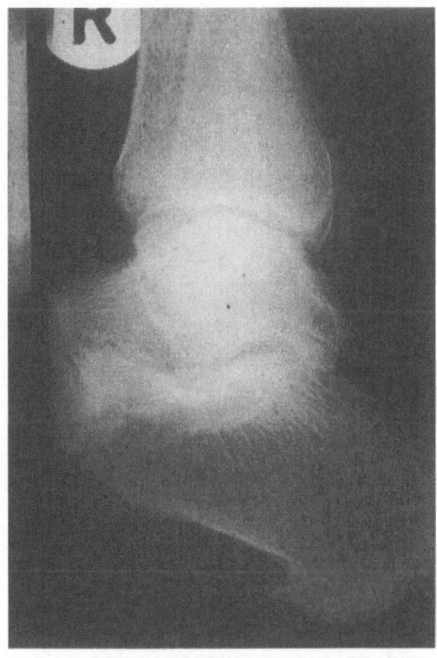

'Spur' on plantar surface in a patient with plantar fasciitis (a result of periosteal inflammation – not sure of the cause of pain)

Figure 6.1

help to alleviate symptoms. Obviously obesity is also a factor which must be corrected.

Occasionally a patient thought to have plantar fasciitis is found to have a chronic or acute lumbar disc lesion and the heel pain and tenderness turns out not to be primary but referred from the spine. There may or may not be a history of sciatica in the S_1 distribution. This condition often responds to lumbar traction.

Panniculitis

The pain of 'fat lady's knee' is often the result of large, tender lumps of adipose tissue surrounding the joint, and is called panniculitis (see Figure 6.2). However, these may occur quite independently away from joints, as for example on the fronts of the legs. Why the fat accumulates in this way and what exactly is the pathological nature of panniculitis is unknown; while patients are occasionally diabetic or hypothyroid, there is no real evidence that the condition is associated with any metab-

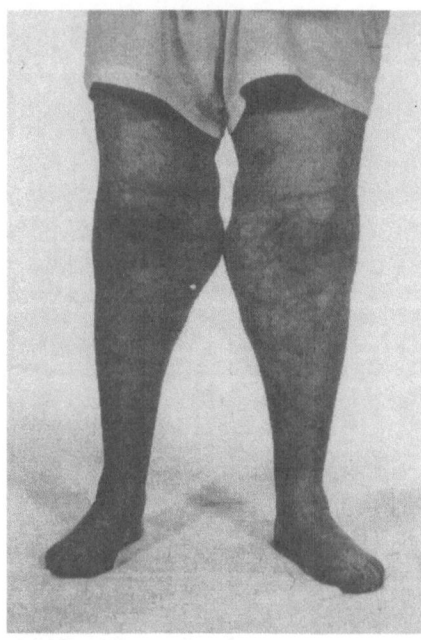

Figure 6.2

'Dewlaps' (panniculins) causing pain on the medial sides of both knees

olic disorder. Treatment is usually ineffectual; acupuncture or ultrasound sometimes help, but only very strict dieting causing profound weight loss influences these fat deposits. A diuretic can occasionally help.

Fibrositis

While strictly denoting inflammation of fibrous tissue, the term 'fibrositis' can mean just about anything. More often than not it implies areas of muscle spasm around the neck, thoracic or lumbar spine which are often related to spondylosis, but X-rays may show only minimal pathology and the condition is often associated with deep-seated anxiety syndromes. Occasionally fibrositis can be set up by calcific deposits deposited in muscle or fascia, either locally (see Figure 6.1) or in generalized chondrocalcinosis. The well-known 'fibrositic nodules' are probably not even composed of fibrous tissue at all but of little balls of muscle spasm; some have been thought to be herniations of fatty lumps through the fascia. There may be vague areas of swelling but basically fibrositis is characterized by tender points in the muscles, and in localizing these it must be remembered that

Fibrositic
nodules

80

several normally tender points exist, such as in the midpoints of the upper surfaces of the trapezius muscles. These normally tender points are thought to be especially tender in fibrositis and may respond to acupuncture.

'Fibrositis syndrome'

A complete 'fibrositis syndrome' has been described, characterized by diffuse pain which is aggravated by fatigue or weather change, stiffness, exhaustion, disturbed sleep, muscle and skinfold tenderness. There is some evidence of relative endorphin deficiency in these patients. Possible treatments include acupuncture, physiotherapy and drugs for anxiety and depression.

Myositis

Polymyositis

The most important type of true myositis is polymyositis – muscle pain and weakness due to both inflammation and degeneration of voluntary muscle. This may be primary or – particularly in elderly people – may be associated with malignant disease elsewhere, so patients must always be fully investigated. Polymyositis is also quite common in certain systemic connective tissue disorders such as systemic sclerosis and some cases of severe rheumatoid arthritis. The diagnosis is suspected clinically, made highly probable by electromyographic changes and elevated serum muscle enzymes, and proven by muscle biopsy.

Fairly large doses of steroid are required for control of primary polymyositis and not all cases respond. Some require immunosuppressive drugs, and often treatment is a matter for the rheumatologist. Isolation of an underlying neoplasm and its successful removal often leads to complete regression of polymyositis.

Polymyalgia rheumatica

Polymyalgic syndrome

This is not a myositis (the muscles are not inflamed or degenerated) but a *syndrome* with many possible causes characterized by pain and stiffness of the proximal muscles (rather than the joints), and mainly affects elderly women who have a high ESR. The classical picture comprises:

(1) Central muscle/joint pain.
(2) Severe, prolonged morning stiffness.
(3) Fatigue and malaise.
(4) High ESR.
(5) Response to small or moderate doses of steroids.

Many patients have a high serum alkaline phosphatase, thought to be due to mild hepatic disturbance, and this is often helpful diagnostically. Polymyalgia usually comes on acutely and untreated remains severe for some months when symptoms gradually ease up, but pain and stiffness can persist for several years before complete recovery occurs, and patients have to remain on small doses of steroid over this period. Some cases of 'fibrositis' are perhaps the aftermath of polymyalgia – a careful history may reveal an almost-forgotten, severe bout of 'rheumatism' some years previously. Although probably a systemic connective tissue disorder, the nature and cause of most cases of polymyalgia is not known. A minority have cranial (temporal) arteritis and have a positive carotid artery biopsy. Some cases are secondary to an underlying severe illness such as malignant tumour of myeloma, some represent the onset of rheumatoid arthritis which in the elderly often starts with shoulder pain and stiffness. Obviously these conditions should be excluded as far as possible before the patient is given steroids (usually prednisolone 15–20 mg/day initially), which produce prompt relief of symptoms. Another important condition to exclude is subacute bacterial endocarditis which may present with symptoms of polymyalgia – here steroids would undoubtedly be disastrous as by causing fluid retention they could overload a weakened myocardium, not to mention their possible effect in causing dissemination of bacteria. It is clear, therefore, that although the general practitioner may well spot polymyalgia and treat it efficiently, a specialist consultation would be wise in all but the most obvious cases.

Treatment of polymyalgia

Tenosynovitis

Inflammation of tendon sheaths is often seen around the hands and wrists, as in de Quervain's disease – tenosynovitis of the common sheath enclosing the extensor pollicis brevis and abductor pollicis longus tendons at the radial side of the wrist. There may or may not be a history of chronic trauma, and some cases are rheumatoid in nature, occasionally gouty. Local pain and tenderness are marked, but swelling may or may not be present. Crepitus may be felt, subjectively by the patient and objectively by the physician, when the tendon moves in its sheath. Pressure on an adjacent nerve may cause an entrapment syndrome, such as a carpal tunnel syndrome resulting from tenosynovitis of the wrist flexors.

Except where chronic and fibrotic, tenosynovitis usually responds to injection of steroid into the tendon sheath; this may be followed by a course of short-wave diathermy or ultrasound. Chronic cases may require surgical freeing of the tendon sheath.

Bursitis

Bursae are either true protrusions of synovial membrane from the joint (such as Baker's cysts behind the knee) or adventitious sacs (such as occur in prepatellar bursitis, known as 'housemaid's knee'). Bursitis may be simply traumatic or may be part of rheumatoid synovitis or gouty arthritis. In the shoulder we recognize a rather uncommon syndrome, acute subdeltoid bursitis, in which there is severe pain and restricted movements and – unlike capsulitis – an immediate and complete response to steroid injection. *(It should be noted that in the United States the terms bursitis and capsulitis of the shoulder are often used synonymously.)*

Enthesopathy

This recently coined term implies inflammation of the tenoperiosteal junction. Besides simple 'soft-tissue' conditions such as tennis elbow and plantar fasciitis (see above), the enthesopathy also applies to lesions affecting ligamentous and muscle attachments in ankylosing spondylitis.

Capsulitis (periarthritis)
This denotes inflammation spreading round the capsule and other soft tissues surrounding the shoulder. It also occasionally affects the hip joint.

Ligamentous strain

This is either traumatic, as in the common strained (or sprained) lateral ligament of the ankle; or secondary to arthritis, as in the 'medial ligament strain' so often seen in osteoarthritis of the knee (see Chapter 13).

Generalized (soft tissue) rheumatism

The aches and pains of influenza and other acute viral illnesses are felt in the muscles – this (along with backache) being the most common 'generalized soft tissue rheumatism'. Rheumatism is often a feature of the acute stage of hepatitis B (associated with Australia antigen) before jaundice appears; here there may be frank arthritis as well. Diffuse rheumatic pain is a feature of systemic connective-tissue disorders such as polyarteritis and systemic lupus erythematosus. The muscular aching often present in hypothyroidism and in osteomalacia is an example of diffuse rheumatism associated with endocrine disorders. Finally, in some neurological disorders such as Parkinsonism and acute polyneuritis (Guillain-Barré syndrome) the patient may complain of diffuse rheumatic pain.

Psychogenic soft-tissue rheumatism

This important subject is discussed in Chapter 3. While 'psychological overlay' often occurs, purely psychological rheumatism is not a common condition and careful thought is needed before a patient is labelled with this condition. Examples of conditions which are often of psychogenic origin are coccygodynia (though many case are referred downwards from lumbar lesions) and xiphisternal pain (though here again, as with all localized pain and tenderness around the neck and chest, one must carefully exclude a primary lesion of the cervical or thoracic spine).

7 Osteoarthritis

Aetiology and pathology – Clinical varieties – Management in family practice – Management in hospital

Osteoarthritis (degenerative joint disease) is the commonest form of joint disease and, along with soft-tissue rheumatism, accounts for the majority of patients with 'rheumatism' appearing at the surgery. It is therefore very important to know about this condition – often untaught (or only touched on) in medical school. Owing to recent knowledge of the aetiology and pathogenesis the rationale of treatment of osteoarthritis is steadily improving.

Aetiology and pathology

Osteoarthritis (OA) is considered either 'primary', or 'secondary' to certain predisposing factors which include fractures near joints, misalignment of joints (such as congenital dislocation of the hip (see Figure 7.1) chronic or recurrent strain on joints (such as in obesity, or when there are repetitive movements involved in work), pre-existing rheumatoid arthritis or gout, haemarthroses (as in haemophilia), excessive joint mobility (as in the hypermobility syndrome) and certain bone disorders such as Paget's disease. More important in practice is the recognition of factors aggravating symptoms, their removal or control being an integral part of treatment. Examples of these are:

Predisposing factors

Aggravating factors

85

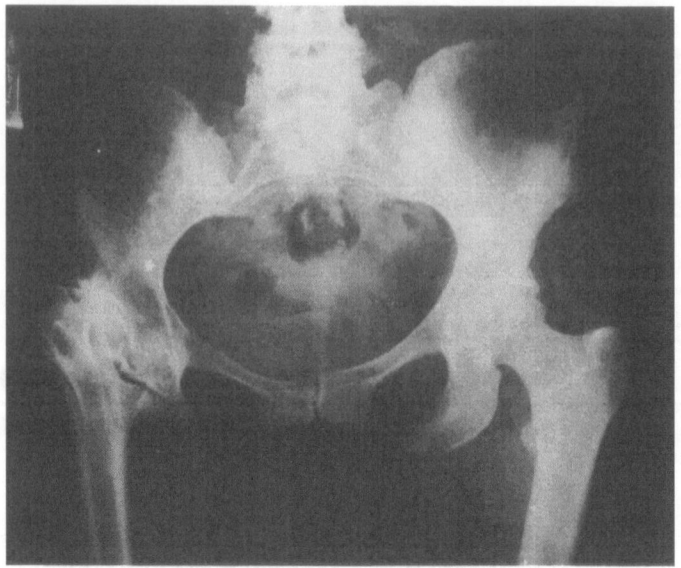

Figure 7.1 Osteoarthritis secondary to congenital dislocation of the right hip

(1) Hypothyroidism.
(2) The menopause and premenstrual syndrome.
(3) Muscle spasm (as in neurological disorders such as in Parkinsonism).
(4) Associated soft-tissue disorders, such as panniculitis and medial ligament strain.
(5) Obesity.
(6) Climate and weather.
(7) Mental upset (anxiety, depression, neurasthenia and hysteria).

Early
pathology

In osteoarthritis the articular cartilage becomes soft and rough and flakes off. Recent work has suggested that in the early stages tiny nodules of calcium apatite crystals are formed within the bone and it is thought that these crystals can be responsible for acute episodes of inflammation in a joint. Later, osteophytes form at the periphery of joints causing the 'lippings' seen in X-rays of the spine and peripheral joints. Finally, in severe cases there is marked loss of cartilage with some destruction of bone, resulting in marked disability.

Clinical varieties

Osteoarthritis may present in one of the following ways:

Presentation
of
osteoarthritis

(1) Pain and stiffness in a large joint; swelling due to synovitis, with or without effusion, may be present.

(2) Pain and stiffness in many joints, small or large. Generalized osteoarthritis, especially in menopausal women, where the terminal interphalangeal (TIP) joints of the fingers, first carpometacarpal joints at the base of the thumbs and the metatarsophalangeal joints of the big toes are most often affected. Patients often have Heberden's nodes adjacent to the terminal interphalangeal joints, occasionally Bouchard's nodes adjacent to the proximal interphalangeal joints of the fingers.

Heberden's
nodes

(3) Spinal pain and stiffness (cervical, thoracic, lumbar spondylosis, or a combination of these).

(4) Symptoms due to a complication, such as paraesthesiae in the medial side of the arm and little and ring fingers due to ulnar nerve entrapment by osteoarthritic changes affecting the ulnar groove of the elbow.

In osteoarthritis involving one or two weight-bearing joints the pain is aggravated by standing or walking. Severe rest and night pain develops as the arthritis becomes more advanced. The synovial fluid aspirated from osteoarthritic effusions is clear and viscid, unless there is associated crystal synovitis when an inflammatory type of fluid may occur. It is stressed again that symptoms of osteoarthritis are often influenced by one or more of the aggravating factors mentioned above.

Management in family practice

Aims of
management

The aims of management are control of pain, improvement of joint mobility, correction of deformity and removal (or at least modification) of aggravating factors.

Control of pain

Analgesics and trial of various anti-inflammatory drugs are always worthwhile. Intra-articular steroids are useful in episodes of acute synovitis, always provided that septic arthritis can be excluded – effusions should always be aspirated, and if cloudy sent for cytology and culture. Steroids are useful

Use of local
steroids in OA

when injected with local anaesthetic into tender adjacent ligaments, such as the medial ligament of the knee in medial ligament strain. Pain is relieved by taking the weight off the joint and by appliances such as splints, lumbar corsets, cervical collars and arch supports (see Chapter 5).

Problems in arthritis and rheumatism

Improvement in joint mobility

Stiffness is helped by exercise therapy and gentle manipulation (especially in spinal osteoarthritis). Exercises preceded by heat treatment also stabilize and strengthen muscles acting on a joint. Stiff, aching finger joints are helped by paraffin wax baths followed by active exercises. Hot wax can also be useful in treating the stiff painful foot, in conjunction with local steroid injections and gentle manipulations.

Correction of deformity

Hospital treatment is required for established deformities of any significance (see below).

Removal of aggravating factors

These have been set out above. Their assessment and removal or modification is usually possible in general practice.

Management in hospital

Reasons for referral — Referral to the rheumatologist or orthopaedic surgeon is often advisable in the following instances:

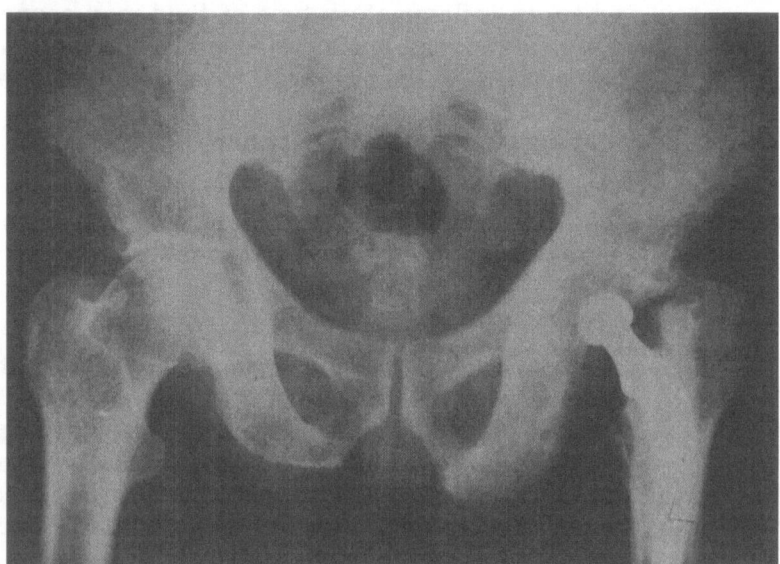

Charnley prosthesis for osteoarthritis of the hip secondary to Paget's disease of the pelvis

Figure 7.2

(1) For aspiration and analysis of joint effusions.
(2) Where specialized physiotherapy or manipulation is required.
(3) For correction or alleviation of deformity, particularly varus, valgus or flexion deformity of the knees. Admission to hospital enables serial splinting, intensive physiotherapy and manipulation under anaesthetic where necessary. Surgery (osteotomy) may be required for correction of severe valgus deformity of the knees.
(4) Surgery may otherwise be required for osteoarthritis of the hip (osteotomy or total hip replacement, see Figure 7.2), arthroplasty of the MTP joint of the big toe and patellofemoral osteoarthritis (patellectomy); when it appears that surgery will be needed the orthopaedic surgeon is often approached, otherwise referral to a rheumatologist is probably advisable in the first instance.

Rheumatoid arthritis

Early recognition – Principal complications – Differential diagnosis – Management of the early case in practice – Hospital management – Rheumatoid arthritis in children and the elderly

Aetiology   For the rheumatologist, rheumatoid arthritis is the big challenge in aetiology diagnosis and treatment. For the family practitioner the main interest centres around (a) early diagnosis – is this patient with joint pain in the process of developing rheumatoid arthritis? – and (b) correct management – what can be done in the surgery, and when should consultant advice be sought?

The cause of rheumatoid disease is still an enigma. More common in females and in middle age, it can, however, occur at any age and of course children are not excluded. Current belief is that some form of infective agent, perhaps a virus, sets up an autoimmune reaction where various forms of antigen–antibody reaction adversely affect not only synovial joints but also many systems, including blood, blood vessels, nerves, muscles and lungs. Cases range from mild, often seronegative instances to severe, highly seropositive, erosive, multisystemic disease.

Early recognition

The possibility of rheumatoid arthritis should be considered in any of the circumstances shown in Table 8.1.

91

Table 8.1   Presenting features of rheumatoid arthritis

Small-joint polyarthritis	insidious pain and swelling (slight or marked) in the small finger joints (especially the proximal interphalangeal and metacarpophalangeal joints, perhaps also the metatarsophalangeal joints of the feet ('like walking on a stone'), usually with considerable morning stiffness.
Large-joint monarthritis	gradual or sudden pain and swelling of one or a few large joints, such as the knees
Acute polyarthritis	sudden pain and swelling of multiple joints, maybe with pyrexia and sweating, often mistaken for rheumatic fever (especially in young patients). *Rheumatic fever is now very rare* and the condition is probably rheumatoid
Persistent tenosynovitis	swollen tendon sheaths, often at the backs of the hands (forming little tense 'lumps') or around the wrists; flexor tenosynovitis may present with paraesthesia in the fingers due to median nerve compression (carpal tunnel syndromes)
Visceral lesion (without arthritis)	a pleural effusion may turn out to be a rheumatoid manifestation before the joints become involved

Confirming the diagnosis

The diagnosis in a suspected case of rheumatoid arthritis (RA) is confirmed by the following steps.

Confirmation
of diagnosis

(1) Examine the patient with care. There may be giveaway signs, such as wrist involvement (unlikely to be due to osteoarthritis as this is rare in the wrists) or tenderness of the lateral metacarpophalangeal joints of the feet (the medial joints are usually involved in osteoarthritis). Look for the following three suggestive features:

(a) Typical deformities (see below).
(b) Palmar erythema (on ulnar sides of the palms – particularly significant in males)
(c) Subcutaneous nodules (in 20–30% cases, especially over backs of the elbows) (see Figure 8.1)

Rheumatoid arthritis

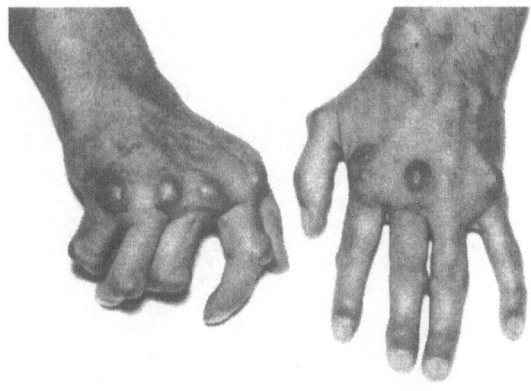

Multiple rheumatoid nodules over the knuckles in rheumatoid arthritis

Figure 8.1

(2) Request a blood count and ESR. There is often a normo-chromic anaemia (see Chapter 3). The ESR is usually *but not always* raised in the early stages.

(3) Request a test for rheumatoid factor (see Chapter 3). The Rose–Waaler and latex tests are often positive, but *not always* in early cases – the test should be repeated 6 months and a year later if symptoms persist. *Note: a negative test for rheumatoid factor does not rule out rheumatoid arthritis.*

(4) If there is a large knee effusion, it should be aspirated – if not by the family doctor then by the rheumatologist. The synovial fluid will have inflammatory features in rheumatoid arthritis (see Chapter 00).

(5) Request X-rays of the hands and feet. Suspicious features are periarticular osteoporosis, periosteal reactions on the phalanges and early erosions (see Figure 8.2).

Consultant referral

Should there still be serious doubt about the diagnosis it is opportune to refer the patient for consultant opinion. In any case many general practitioners like confirmation of their diagnosis, and of course patients, knowing the implications of this diagnosis, may well wish to have another opinion. They should be reassured that there is much one can do to alleviate symptoms and prevent the development of deformities, and that given an acceptable standard of medical treatment, the disease can be reasonably well controlled except in only a small proportion of patients.

93

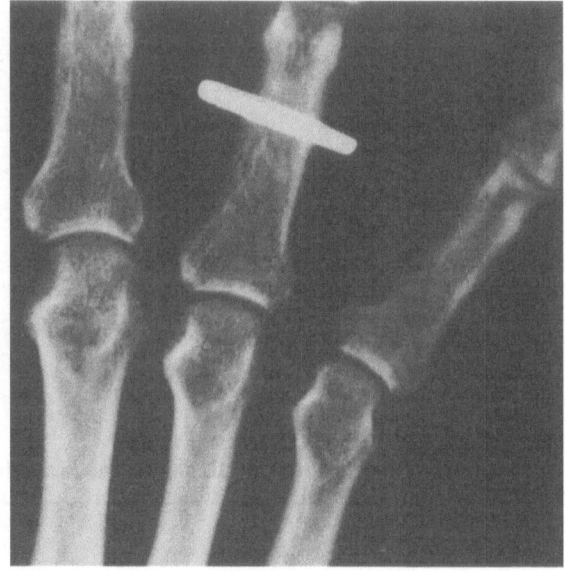

Erosion in the proximal interphalangeal joint of the little finger in a patient with early rheumatoid arthritis

Figure 8.2

Principal complications

In established rheumatoid arthritis the following features and complications may develop as shown in Table 8.2.

Table 8.2   Complications of rheumatoid arthritis

Deformities	for example, ulnar deviation of the MCP joints of the fingers with anterior subluxation of the metacarpals on the phalanges (see Figure 8.3), swan neck deformities characterized by hyper-extension of proximal interphalangeal and flexion of terminal interphalangeal joints of the fingers
Vasculitis	causing skin ulceration or areas of necrosis or gangrene (Figure 8.4)
Muscle wasting and general loss of weight	
Stiffness of joints with loss of normal range of movements	
Cervical spine problems	neck pain, brachial neuralgia, occasionally long tract signs (paraparesis) due to vertebral subluxations (especi-

Table 8.2 (Cont'd)

	ally atlanto-occipital) causing nerve-root or spinal cord pressure.
Eye problems	especially scleritis and keratoconjunctivitis sicca.
Pericarditis and pleurisy	may be a direct manifestation of rheumatoid arthritis; other pulmonary lesions (such as interstitial fibrosis), grouped together as 'rheumatoid lung', may occur
Neuropathy	motor, sensory, sensorimotor or 'entrapment' neuropathies
Anaemia	moderate normochromic anaemia is common and its degree usually relates to the activity of the disease; macrocytic anaemia is rare and may be due to nutritional folic acid deficiency (especially in the elderly), malabsorption or occasionally pernicious anaemia
Amyloid disease	a serious complication of severe rheumatoid arthritis. It should be considered in patients 'going downhill'; it may present with persistent proteinuria and cause a nephrotic syndrome

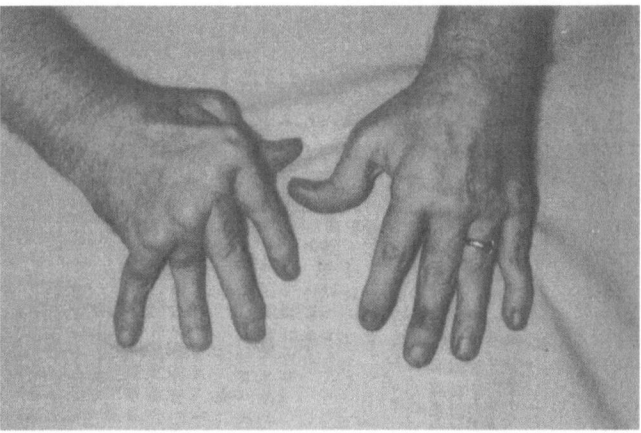

Ulnar deviation of fingers of right hand in a patient with rheumatoid arthritis

Figure 8.3

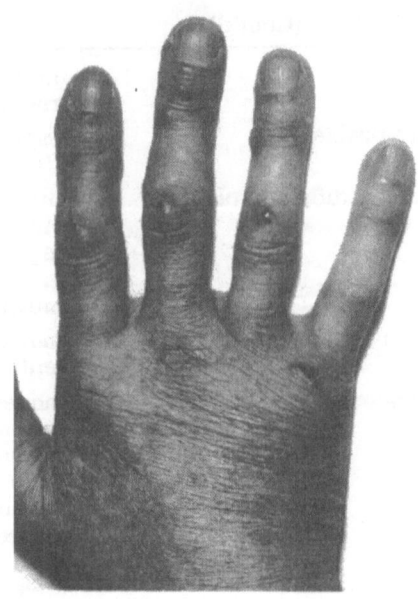

Necrotic skin lesions in a patient with rheumatoid arthritis complicated by arteritis (vasculitis)

Figure 8.4

Differential diagnosis

The following conditions are some of those important in the differential diagnosis of rheumatoid arthritis:

Osteoarthritis

Different small joints are involved (see Chapter 7), and there are Heberden's nodes as opposed to rheumatoid nodules; morning stiffness is absent or of very short duration, and rheumatoid factor is absent.

Virus polyarthritis or arthralgia

The arthritis is usually shortlived, the joints are not very swollen, the ESR is often normal, and rheumatoid factor is absent.

Systemic connective tissue disorders

Systemic lupus erythematosus (SLE), systemic sclerosis and polyarteritis may present with rheumatoid-like features but there is usually marked systemic upset – out of proportion to the joint symptoms – and there are often other specific features (such as the rash of SLE). While rheumatoid factor may be present there are other immunological disorders, such as antinuclear antibody, LE cells and antiDNA antibodies in SLE.

Atypical gout

Occasionally gout presents with an acute polyarthritis or large-joint monarthritis which resembles rheumatoid arthritis. In postpubertal males and postmenopausal females a serum uric acid (SUA) should be a routine investigation, remembering that the SUA may be raised in any patient taking small regular doses of aspirin or diuretics.

Acute septic arthritis

This usually involves just one joint. This is hot, extremely painful and swollen, and there is marked pyrexia. The diagnosis is established by withdrawing purulent synovial fluid and finding pyogenic bacteria either by direct examination or after culture.

Reactive arthritis

Reiter's syndrome, rheumatic fever and other forms of reactive arthritis may be mistaken for rheumatoid arthritis.

Seronegative HLA-B27 associated arthritis

The peripheral joints may be involved in ankylosing spondylitis, in psoriatic arthritis (which may exist in the absence of current psoriasis) and in the arthritis or arthralgia associated with ulcerative colitis or Crohn's disease.

Management of the early case in practice

Patients with early rheumatoid arthritis can often be adequately treated by the general practitioner provided certain basic principles are kept in mind. Occasionally admission to hospital is required, particularly in very acute or complicated cases. It is advisable to consult a rheumatologist for guidance in treatment when there is no adequate response following simple regime.

Basic management of early rheumatoid arthritis

The following six steps should be observed initially.

(1) Rest: if possible, rest in bed for a week or two.
(2) Analgesics: see Chapter 5.
(3) Salicylates: it is still good practice to prescribe aspirin or aspirin derivatives in full dosage in the initial treatment.
(4) Non-steroidal anti-inflammatory drugs: see Chapter 5.
(5) Intra-articular steroid injections: one or a few persistently active joints may be injected; see Chapter 5.
(6) Convalescence: after rheumatoid activity has subsided a holiday is advisable, and there should certainly be a reasonable period before work is recommenced.

The hospital management of rheumatoid arthritis
Basic principles of management

There are ten basic principles of management of the established case of rheumatoid arthritis. Many of these entail hospital attendance as an outpatient, if not admission.

(1) Alleviation of pain.
(2) Rest, mental and physical (if necessary in hospital).
(3) Reduction of generalized rheumatoid activity.
(4) Reduction of activity in individual joints.
(5) Improvement in mobility and function of joints.
(6) Correction of deformities.
(7) Improvement of general health.
(8) Treatment of intercurrent disease.
(9) Treatment of complications.
(10) Education of the patient.

For a detailed discussion of these the reader is referred to the various sections of Chapter 5 and to the author's recent textbook (Golding, 1979). Following are some comments on aspects of these problems which are of interest to general practitioners.

Alleviation of pain
Alleviation of pain is achieved by rest, splinting active joints, analgesic and anti-inflammatory drugs and intra-articular and soft-tissue steroid injections (see Chapter 6).

Treatment of generalized rheumatoid activity
Generalized rheumatoid activity is reduced by rest, splinting of several joints and anti-inflammatory drugs (which include non-steroidal anti-inflammatory drugs (NSAID) and systemic corticosteroids, described in Chapter 6), immunosuppressive

drugs (also described in Chapter 6 and the specific anti-rheum-atoid drugs (such as gold, penicillamine and chloroquine) which are described below. The progression of use of these drugs is as shown in Table 8.3.

Table 8.3 Use of anti-inflammatory drugs

Start with
Aspirin (high-dose) or perhaps Ketoprofen
↓
Non-steroidal anti-inflammatory drugs (NSAID)
↓
Specific anti-rheumatoid drugs
(gold, penicillamine, chloroquine)
↓   or   ↓
Systemic steroids   Immunosuppressive agents

Activity in individual joints

Activity in individual joints is reckoned by aspiration of effusions, injection of steroid, resting the joints (as by avoiding weight-bearing or splinting the joints), 'medical synovectomy' by injecting radioactive colloids such as yttrium 90, or (surgical) synovectomy.

Improvement of mobility and function

Improvement of mobility and function of joints as described in Chapter 5 includes exercise therapy, hydrotherapy, specific occupational therapy and certain surgical procedures including (in advanced cases) prosthetic replacement of joints.

Correction of deformities

Correction of deformities may be achieved by serial splinting of joints, physiotherapy or surgery.

Specific anti-rheumatoid drugs

Specific drugs

These are drugs which have an anti-inflammatory effect specifically in rheumatoid arthritis (but not other forms of arthritis) and which perhaps favourably influence the cause of the disease; they are indicated where disease activity persists in spite of rest, splinting, steroid injections and nonsteroidal anti-inflammatory drugs. The exact point at which such drugs are introduced varies amongst rheumatologists. Some prefer to introduce gold or penicillamine at a relatively early stage of the disease, others persist with 'conservative treatment' for a longer period. Most practitioners would try one of these drugs before resorting to systemic steroids, though some prefer to try immunosuppressive drugs first. Both gold and penicillamine have been shown to be effective in a high proportion of rheumatoid patients, and the titre of rheumatoid factor often drops

Gold and penicillamine

Chloroquine

together with clinical improvement. Chloroquine is less potent and less often used, but may return to favour in less severe cases and perhaps in children with seropositive disease.

Penicillamine

Penicillamine is prescribed in the 'go slow, go low' manner, starting with 125 mg/day or perhaps 250 mg/day for a few weeks, increasing to 500 mg/day if necessary, occasionally 750 mg/day but not more. At least a month (often 6–8 weeks) elapses before its action is apparent. Penicillamine and gold therapy must be monitored by carrying out the following tests at 2-weekly intervals:

(1) Blood count, including platelet count
(2) Urine test, for albumin and blood

Thrombo-cytopenia and albuminuria

These tests are essential to observe progressive thrombocytopenia or albuminuria, either of which may require withdrawal of the drug. Other important side-effects of penicillamine are severe loss of taste, rashes (early hypersensitivity rashes are of little importance but rarely pemphigoid and exfoliative dermatitis may occur) and (very rarely) a myasthenic syndrome.

Gold

Gold has a similar action to penicillamine. Myocrisin (sodium aurothiomalate) is given by intramuscular injection, starting with 'test' injections of 10 and 20 mg (for allergy) and then 50 mg weekly to a total dose of 500 mg (some continue to 1 g). Maintenance injections of 50 mg every month may be continued, but there is little evidence that continuous gold therapy is advantageous. As with penicillamine, 2-weekly or at least monthly screening is essential to detect neutropenia, thrombocytopenia and nephropathy. Gold can cause severe exfoliative dermatitis, stomatitis and corneal ulceration. Oral gold preparations are now under trial.

Disadvantages of gold therapy

Chloroquine

The main drawback of chloroquine and other antimalarial drugs is the potential hazard of retinopathy, which may cause blindness if severe and progressive. However, this is most unlikely if the drug is prescribed in short courses of 6–9 months using small doses (250–500 mg day chloroquine phosphate). It is still wise to ask an ophthalmologist to screen the eyes before starting chloroquine, after starting the drug and then at intervals of a few months.

Rheumatoid arthritis in children and the elderly

Various forms of 'rheumatism' and 'growing pains' are common in *childhood*, but true inflammatory arthritis is fortunately

100

uncommon. Cases of suspected arthritis should be referred to a consultant rheumatologist as assessment and diagnosis is often difficult.

Juvenile chronic arthritis (JCA)

Juvenile chronic arthritis may be one of several varieties:

Varieties of juvenile chronic arthritis

(1) Seropositive ('adult type') rheumatoid arthritis – systemic (Still's disease)

(2) Seronegative JCA – polyarthritis; oligoarticular (affecting a few joints); monarticular.

(3) Seronegative HLA-B27 associated arthritis, usually with sacroiliitis (though the radiological diagnosis is very difficult in childhood) and sometimes progressive to true ankylosing spondylitis in adolescence or early adulthood.

(4) Miscellaneous disorders, such as leukaemic arthritis.

Still's disease

Still's disease and other forms of seronegative JCA often differ from adult type rheumatoid arthritis in the frequency of involvement of certain joints, such as the cervical spine: the presence of radiological sacroiliitis; absence of subcutaneous nodules; general and local growth disturbances; rash, fever and lymphadenopathy (in classical Still's disease); frequent eye lesions (iritis and keratitis – all children with arthritis should be screened by slitlamp examination).

Arthritis in the elderly

Elderly sufferers

At the other end of the age-spectrum it is not unusual for rheumatoid arthritis to appear for the first time in elderly patients. The disease is often relatively mild and responds well to conservative treatment with a good prognosis. A common mode of onset is pain and stiffness in the shoulders, the clinical picture resembling polymyalgia rheumatica which is often diagnosed in error. In the treatment of arthritis in the elderly there is: (1) the tendency to deafness and tinnitus when salicylates are given, even in small doses; (2) the frequency of side-effects with certain non-steroidal anti-inflammatory drugs, such as indomethacin (naproxen is a much more acceptable drug in the elderly); (3) the inadvisability of gold and penicillamine therapy because of the frequency of renal dysfunction in old people. Should there not be an adequate response to conservative treatment, such as physiotherapy and steroid injections, small doses of systemic prednisolone should be seriously considered at a relatively early stage as the risk of serious side-effects in the future is less important in this age-group.

Ankylosing spondylitis and seronegative spondarthritis

Concept of seronegative spondarthritis – Clinical features – Ankylosing spondylitis: Management in practice

Ankylosing spondylitis is an important cause of back pain in young persons. It is an inflammatory type of arthritis of the spine and sacroiliac joints, a rheumatoid-like condition of the spine. In fact, it was once actually thought to be rheumatoid arthritis of the spine; we now know that this is not so – rheumatoid factor is **Ankylosing** not present in ankylosing spondylitis, the peripheral joints are **spondylitis** *vs.* not usually involved (though they are occasionally) and the pain **rheumatoid** responds in a curiously brisk and almost 'specific' manner to **arthritis** deep X-ray therapy and anti-inflammatory drugs. Ankylosing spondylitis is one of a group of conditions known as *seronegative spondarthritis* (a division of seronegative arthritis in general) – see Table 9.1.

Table 9.1   Classification of seronegative arthritis

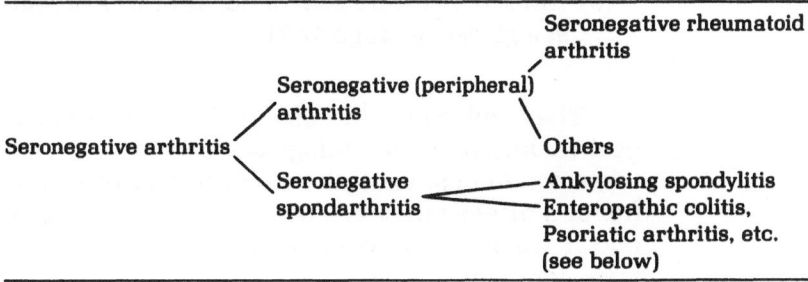

Concept of seronegative spondarthritis

Sacroiliitis

Patients with seronegative spondarthritis primarily have inflammatory disease of the spinal and sacroiliac joints and sometimes there is peripheral arthritis as well. The main clinical and radiological feature is sacroiliitis, inflammation leading to erosion, irregularity and sometimes ankylosis of one or both sacroiliac joints. There is much clinical overlap between the various conditions comprising this group of conditions, which tend to show familial aggregation and have in common a high prevalence of the histocompatibility antigen HLA-B27 (see Chapter 3) which can be a valuable diagnostic marker in doubtful cases.

The main varieties of seronegative spondarthritis

These are:

(1) Ankylosing spondylitis
(2) Psoriatic arthritis   ⎧ in ulcerative colitis
(3) Enteropathic arthritis ⎨ in Crohn's disease
(4) Reiter's disease   ⎩ in Whipple's disease

From this it will be clear that, in addition to spinal X-rays, basic investigations required in a patient found to have sacroiliitis (and indeed in any patient who has atypical, persistently seronegative arthritis) will be:

Sacroiliitis: investigations

(1) Blood-count and ESR
(2) HLA antigens
(3) Search for psoriasis (and enquiry for psoriasis in any close relative)
(4) Barium meal/barium enema/ sigmoidoscopy
(5) MSU, GCFT (and search for features of Reiter's disease – see glossary, page 147).

The reader should consult the glossary at the end of this book (or larger rheumatology textbooks) for the main features of these conditions. With the exception of psoriatic arthritis and Reiter's disease they are not very common in general practice, and it would be wise to refer suspected cases for specialist investigation.

Ankylosing spondylitis – clinical features

It is very important to recognize ankylosing spondylitis because early treatment, that is, simply anti-inflammatory drugs and spinal exercises, can prevent future deformity and minimize spinal stiffness. It commonly affects young men, and occasionally females. How can we decide that a young man with back pain has this condition? It is helpful to remember ten suggestive features:

Features suggestive of ankylosing spondylitis

(1) There is often a family history of the condition.

(2) The pain may be situated over the buttocks, that is, the sacroiliac joints, but it can be central – in the spine. Pain originating in the thoracic spine may radiate around the chest and cause apparent dyspnoea.

(3) There is usually marked morning stiffness affecting the spine which lasts more than 30 minutes.

(4) Occasionally there is peripheral joint involvement, especially the large joints such as the knees.

(5) There is often a history of attacks of iritis (anterior uveitis) – sometimes the first attack of iritis is coincidental with the first episode of back pain.

(6) Examination of the back shows marked stiffness in all planes.

(7) It is worth auscultating the heart for an aortic murmur. While a rare event, aortic incompetence is a characteristic lesion of spondylitis and can therefore be helpful diagnostically.

(8) The X-ray will usually show features of sacroiliitis – indistinct, slightly irregular sacroiliac joints – but definite changes are often lacking in early cases. Coned and oblique views of the sacroiliac joints may be helpful. The important early spinal feature is the syndesmophyte – a bridge of new bone connecting two vertebrae in a vertical direction (as opposed to the horizontal direction of osteophytes in spinal osteoarthritis).

(9) The ESR may be raised, but this is not always the case – a *normal ESR does not refute the diagnosis.*

(10) The presence of HLA-B27 lends weight to the diagnosis, but does not prove it, as the antigen is present in 7% of normal people.

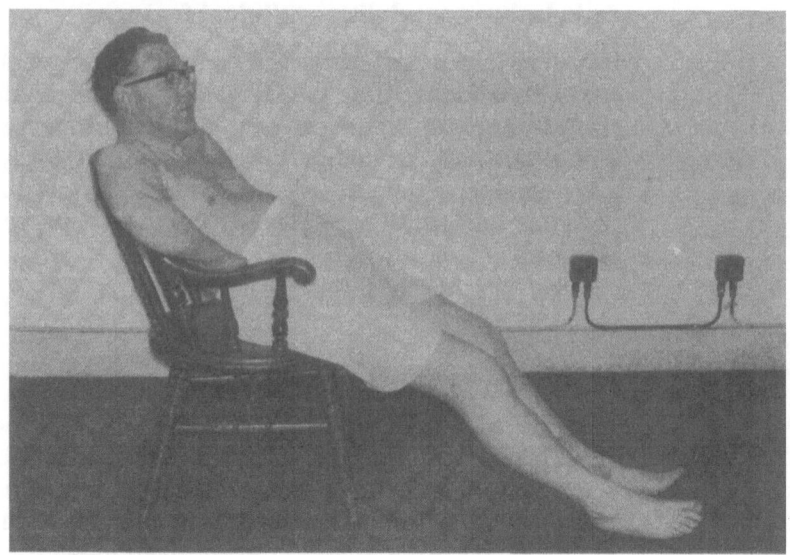

Rigid spine and hips in a patient with advanced ankylosing spondylitis
who was unable to sit comfortably in a chair

Figure 9.1

Advanced ankylosing spondylitis

The patient with advanced ankylosing spondylitis, with the
characteristic stoop and rigid spine ('poker back') and ligamentous calcification in the X-ray, is easy to recognize. Even though
deformity can be prevented by early treatment, there is a possibility of functional handicap from progressive involvement of
the hips (fortunately, now correctable by total hip replacement)
– an example is shown in Figure 9.1 – from progressive immobil-
ity of the neck so that the patient is unable to look round and is
thereby at risk when driving or even just crossing the road or
from fractures and dislocations of cervical vertebrae with the
risk of spinal cord injury.

Active and inactive phases

As in rheumatoid arthritis there are active and inactive phases
in ankylosing spondylitis, disease activity being judged on the
degree of pain, duration of morning stiffness and the ESR.
Occasionally patients with very active disease are ill, lose
weight and show severe constitutional symptoms requiring a
period of intensive hospital treatment. Otherwise, most patients
can usually be managed by their own family physician and do
not need to attend a hospital outpatient department regularly.

Management in general practice

We are mainly concerned with the early or recently recognized case. The two main items in treatment are (a) relief of pain by non-steroidal anti-inflammatory drugs, and (b) improvement of spinal mobility.

Relief of pain by anti-inflammatory drugs

The pain of spondylitis is often dramatically relieved by anti-inflammatory drugs and indeed this rapid response can be diagnostically helpful. Small doses of phenylbutazone appear to be as good as any and can be tried first – some patients need to take only 100 mg once or twice daily, or even just a few tablets per week. There is often an equally good response to indomethacin, flurbiprofen or any of the other agents (see Chapter 5). But, except for the most fulminant cases when short courses of systemic steroids may be prescribed, these are not required, are often disappointing in their effect and indeed can be dangerous in the long run owing to the risk of progressive loss of calcium from the vertebrae, which may well be already osteoporotic. (*Note:* while deep X-ray therapy is often effective this treatment has been virtually abandoned owing to the potential risk of eventual blood dyscrasias.)

Improvement of spinal mobility

Exercise therapy

When pain is totally or at least largely relieved the patient is given a comprehensive list of daily exercises to mobilize all sections of the spine. Especially where there is extensive spinal involvement a preliminary course of exercises in the hydrotherapy pool is useful and the patient is encouraged to swim regularly. In all cases regular exercises are imperative, including those to improve posture while sitting, standing and walking, and breathing exercises to improve respiratory ventilation.

Other aspects of treatment

Other aspects of treatment that may need to be considered in certain cases are: *aspiration of knee effusions* when they occur, *total hip replacement* for progressive ankylosis of the hips, *local steroid injections* for peripheral arthritis and soft-tissue lesions such as plantar fasciitis. Patient education (including genetic counselling) is important. Sometimes modification or occasionally complete change of work is required.

Importance of patient education

10 Gout and crystal deposition arthritis

Crystal deposition arthritis: clinical varieties – Gout: investigation of patients – Treatment of gout – Investigation and treatment of chondrocalcinosis

Crystal deposition disease

Chondro-calcinosis

Certain types of joint pain, effusions and arthritis are now recognized to be a result of crystal deposition in the synovial membrane. Apparently the crystals attract immunoglobulins to their negatively charged surfaces and thereby initiate an inflammatory reaction in the joint. While most cases of chondrocalcinosis are idiopathic, we are beginning to discover a metabolic or endocrine basis for the deposition of these crystals. Of course, it has been known for some time that urate crystals, formed as a result of hyperuricaemia – either as a primary metabolic error in which excessive uric acid is formed or secondary to excessive production or insufficient excretion of urate – are responsible for gouty attacks. More recently, various types of arthritis due to deposition of calcium salts have been recognized; the acute varieties which very much resemble classical gout are called pseudogout.

Crystal deposition arthritis: clinical varieties

At the present time the following disorders of joints are recognized as being a result of crystal deposition:

(1) Classical acute gout (urate crystals).
(2) Atypical gout (such as, polyarthritis, knee effusions) (urate crystals).

109

(3) Chronic tophaceous gout (tophi formed by urate crystals together with a granulomatous reaction).

(4) Pseudogout (acute chondrocalcinosis) (pyrophosphate crystals).

(5) Chronic arthritis with chondrocalcinosis (pyrophosphate crystals).

(6) Chronic destructive arthritis (pyrophosphate crystals).

} Chondrocalcinosis

(7) Acute calcific tendinitis (periarthritis – the calcified rotator cuff lesion of the shoulder) (hydroxyapatite crystals).

(8) Some episodes of acute synovitis in osteoarthritic joints (see Chapter 9) (hydroxyapatite crystals).

Classical acute gout

Acute gout

This needs no description; it is probably more familiar to the general practitioner than the rheumatologist. The attacks of pain, redness and swelling in the big toe spreading up the foot last 2–4 days but may go on for 2 weeks unless treated with an anti-inflammatory drug. The possibility of gout as a cause of acute arthritis in joints other than the metatarsophalangeal joint of the big toe must be remembered in any case of acute monarthritis, but in addition to chondrocalcinosis rheumatoid arthritis, psoriatic arthritis and others may present in this manner. The serum uric acid is usually, though not invariably, elevated during the acute attack of gout and more than one SUA should be requested.

Elevated SUA in gout

Atypical gout

The type that may cause recurrent pain and effusion in the knees can be difficult to diagnose, unless synovial fluid is aspirated and urate crystals found in a fresh specimen. The fluid often appears highly 'inflammatory' – turbid and non-viscous, with a high cell count – but this is not always the case.

Chronic tophaceous gout

This is becoming quite uncommon because of early diagnosis and treatment with allopurinol. Cysts containing urate appear

Tophi in the phalanges and may become very large and irregular with thin walls. Tophi are hard, irregular swellings around the joints which ulcerate, releasing a chalky material composed of urate with calcium oxalate.

Pseudogout (acute chondrocalcinosis)

This often affects the knees, but other joints such as the wrists and also the spine may be involved. X-rays show linear calcification of articular cartilage and menisci (see Figure 10.1) the joint fluid appears inflammatory and typical pyrophosphate crystals are found by examination with polarized light microscopy.

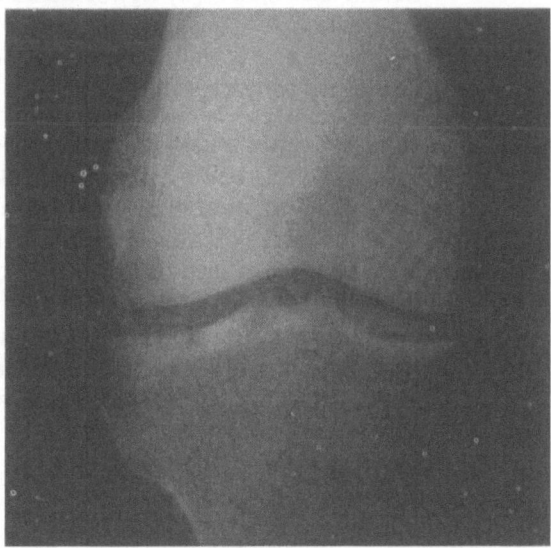

Calcified articular cartilage in the knee joint of a patient with chondrocalcinosis

Figure 10.1 _____

Chronic arthritis with chondrocalcinosis

This is usually a degenerative joint disorder (secondary form of osteoarthritis). Rarely, a severe, destructive arthritis resembling a neuropathic joint is a result of frequent acute attacks.

Gout: investigation of patients

The essential investigation of gout includes:

111

(1) Noting family history.
(2) Estimation of serum uric acid estimations.
(3) Taking a blood count (myeloproliferative disorders such as leukaemia and reticuloses may lead to secondary gout).
(4) Measuring blood urea and creatinine (renal failure is a cause of hyperuricaemia; long-standing hyperuricaemia can lead to renal insufficiency).
(5) Noting current drug therapy (diuretics especially, small doses of aspirin, and anithypertensive agents such as mecamylamine, can induce hyperuricaemia and may precipitate gout in a patient predisposed to it).
(6) Measuring serum calcium, phosphorus and alkaline phosphatase. (hyperparathyroidism may lead to (a) hyperuricaemia and gout, (b) hypercalcaemia and pyrophosphate arthritis).
(7) Where there is an effusion, aspirating synovial fluid and examining for crystals.

Age and sex in gout

Note: pre-menopausal women never (or hardly ever) get gout. The same is true of prepubertal children, except in the extremely rare instance of the Lesch–Nyhan syndrome, an inherited metabolic disease in which there is also neurological disorder and mental deficiency.

Alcohol in gout

Patients often ask whether overindulgence in alcoholic beverage causes gout. This is not the case, although an alcoholic binge may precipitate an attack, as alcohol raises the blood lactic acid, inducing retention of urate by the kidneys.

Treatment of gout
Acute attacks

When a patient is seen in an acute attack the limb is propped up, rested, cooled and protected from the bedclothes (every little stimulus is excruciatingly painful). Large doses of a non-steroidal anti-inflammatory drug (such as phenylbutazone 300 mg t.i.d. or indomethacin 100 mg t.i.d.) are given for a day or two by which time the attack will often have almost subsided, the drug being tailed off over the next few days. (*Note:* allopurinol is *not* given in the acute state, only to prevent acute attacks.) Joint effusions are aspirated and sent for culture (to exclude septic arthritis) and crystal identification.

Phenylbutazone and indomethacin

Preventing acute attacks

To prevent further attacks, having excluded a primary cause for

Allopurinol   hyperuricaemia the patient is given allopurinol 300 mg as a single morning dose and the serum uric acid level is monitored. For the first few weeks of allopurinol therapy small doses of an anti-inflammatory drug are also given, otherwise a sudden influx of urate from the tissues into the blood can lead to an acute attack. Allopurinol prevents uric acid synthesis, as the serum uric acid becomes normal in most patients and gouty attacks cease. Occasionally a larger dose of allopurinol is required to normalize the serum uric acid. Very occasionally the condition is resistant to allopurinol when another uricosuric agent (such as probenecid) is used – here the advice of a rheum-

Diet in gout   atologist may be required. Diet is no longer important in treatment; before the advent of uric acid-lowering drugs patients were advised to drastically reduce their intake of foods containing nucleoprotein (from which uric acid is derived), but this is no longer necessary.

Investigation and treatment of chondrocalcinosis (pseudogout)

While it is not usual to discover a metabolic basis for chondro-calcinosis the following tests should be carried out to exclude certain conditions:

(1) Serum uric acid (to exclude urate gout which may accompany chondrocalcinosis)
(2) Serum calcium, phosphorus and alkaline phosphatase (to exclude hyperparathyroidism). If these are abnormal the advice of a rheumatologist should be sought to advise on further investigation into the possibility of a parathyroid tumour.
(3) Serum iron and iron-building capacity (to exclude haemachrometosis).

Treatment of   Unless an underlying metabolic abnormality is detected, other than aspiration of effusions, the treatment of pseudogout

pseudogout   is non-specific, and the condition responds quite well to non-steroidal anti-inflammatory drugs. Chronic chondrocalcinosis with secondary osteoarthritis often requires vigorous physiotherapy to mobilize and keep mobile a joint which is prone to become very stiff. Sometimes steroid injections help, especially given into the medial ligaments of the knees, as described under the treatment of osteoarthritis.

SECTION 3
Regional Pain Syndromes

11 Pain in the neck and back

Common causes of pain – Investigation of neck pain syndromes – Treatment of neck pain syndromes – Investigation of low back pain – Treatment of low back pain.

Common causes of pain

The most common causes of pain in the neck and back are traumatic and degenerative lesions of the intervertebral discs and the small joints articulating between the vertebral bodies and arches (known as the apophyseal joints).

Very common causes are:

(1) Degenerative lesions of the discs and small articulating (apophyseal) joints. This is called cervical and lumbar spondylosis (osteoarthritis).
(2) Traumatic lesions of the above, often in discs and joints already 'weakened' by spondylosis.

Much less commonly, neck or back pain is due to:

(3) A fracture of a vertebra or neural arch.
(4) Soft-tissue and ligamentous sprains.
(5) Postural abnormalities (such as drooping shoulder-girdles, long-standing kyphosis) excessive lordosis.
(6) Hypermobility (the 'loose back syndrome').
(7) Ankylosing spondylitis (or other forms of sacroiliitis).
(8) Infections (including tuberculosis).
(9) Neoplasms (usually secondary).

(10) Metabolic bone disease (usually osteomalacia or severe osteoporosis).
(11) Paget's disease of the vertebrae or pelvis.
(12) Tumours and other disorders of the spinal cord.

Though uncommon, it is clearly essential to recognize causes (6) to (12) above.

Aggravation of backache

Backache can be aggravated by postural strain, shortening of one leg (as in osteoarthritis of the hip), congenital defects of the vertebrae such as sacralization of L_5 (especially if this is unilateral) or spondylolisthesis (backward or forward slipping of one vertebrae on another – sometimes congenital with a break in the pars interarticularis, sometimes due to degenerative joint disease).

Secondary effects

Besides local spinal pain, secondary effects of disc lesions and spondylosis include the following:

(1) Nerve-root pressure (sciatica or brachial neuralgia and paraesthesiae in root distribution).
(2) Referred pain around chest wall (from thoracic lesions).
(3) Vertebral artery compression (in cervical lesions, giving attacks of 'vertebro-basilar ischaemia' with dizziness on moving the neck).
(4) Spinal cord pressure (giving leg weakness from an upper motor neurone lesion).
(5) Neurogenic claudication (resembling vascular intermittent claudication, due to a lumbar disc lesion but often associated with spinal stenosis).

Investigation of neck pain syndromes

In patients with neck pain (with or without brachial neuralgia) routine clinical examination should include neck movements in all directions, neurological examination of the arms and legs and careful search for local tenderness over and around the cervical spine. The physicians should attempt to differentiate a true 'block' of neck movements in one or more directions from general stiffness due to painful muscle spasm.

Cervical spine X-rays   Radiographs of the cervical spine often show 'cervical spondylosis' and disc narrowing but it is difficult to assess the significance of these findings, particularly in older patients where degenerative changes are ubiquitious. *Clinical assessment is much more important.* X-rays are needed where rheumatoid arthritis involves the neck, in ankylosing spondylosis, in suspected malignant disease, and whenever the pain does not respond to standard treatment.

Treatment of neck pain syndromes

The following facts should be borne in mind when planning treatment for patients with neck pain due to disc lesions or cervical spondylosis:

(1) Often the symptoms are recurrent, with periods of exacerbation and remission each lasting about 3 months.
(2) Where muscle spasm is clearly prominent, this should receive attention (by muscle relaxant drugs or perhaps acupuncture).
(3) As already mentioned, there may also be a thoracic spine lesion, symptoms often summating with those due to the cervical lesion; both levels require treatment.
(4) Admission to hospital is often required for cases with evidence of spinal cord pressure – sometimes immobilization in a firm collar suffices.
(5) Whereas the rheumatoid cervical spine must be *immobilized* in a strong collar, in ankylosing spondylitis there should be an attempt at *mobilizing* the neck by exercise therapy.

    The average case of cervical pain with brachial neuralgia is initially treated by resting the neck in a soft collar and prescribing analgesics and muscle relaxant drugs such as diazepam. Where pain in the arm (brachial neuralgia) is a feature intermittent neck traction is prescribed later on – this should be given at least three times weekly. Should the neck remain stiff a gentle manipulation may be tried and this is supplemented with a course of Maitland manipulations carried out by the physiotherapist. Finally, graduated exercise therapy is introduced and – most importantly – the patient is taught to Need for admission to hospital continue the neck exercises at home. Where brachial neuralgia persists, admission to hospital for further investigation, perhaps including cervical myelography, and continuous neck trac-

119

tion, is required. Only very occasionally is surgical treatment (cervical fusion with decompression of the nerve root) needed.

Investigation of low back pain

Examination

Routine examination in a patient with low back pain includes inspection of the back for deformity while standing, assessment of back movements, straight-leg raising (limitation indicates a lower lumbar lesion), femoral nerve stretch (if painful this indicates an upper lumbar lesion), neurological examination of the legs and palpation of the spine for local tenderness.

X-rays in back pain

Radiographs are advisable in severe and persistent cases. As in the cervical region, evidence of 'spondylosis' is not to be taken too seriously unless (a) there are one or more localized degenerative disc lesions which correspond to the level of pain or root involvement, or (b) osteoarthritis is evident in the posterior apophyseal joints (as opposed to the discs or vertebrae) – this can be responsible for intractable backache, or (c) there is gross anterior spondylosis (large osteophytes) which may catch an emerging nerve root. When anterior spondylosis is severe

Senile ankylosing hyperostosis

(often in the elderly) the condition is known as '(senile) ankylosing hyperostosis'. X-rays may reveal spondylolisthesis (see Figure 11.1), other congenital defects, crush fractures in osteoporosis,

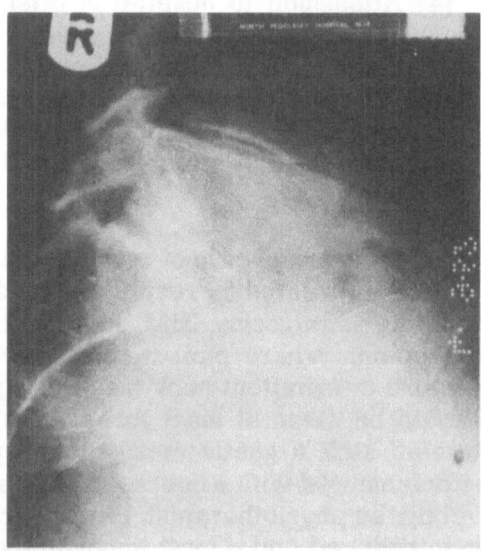

Spondylolisthesis of L4 on L5 with narrowed disc space in a patient with severe backache

Figure 11.1

120

Paget's disease or other bone disorders. Many upper lumbar lesions in elderly patients turn out to be diseases of bone, such as secondary neoplasms; should this be suspected an ESR and phosphatases should be requested. Isotopic scanning of the spine can detect bone tumours even before they are radiologically apparent. However, the interpretation of a bone-scan is often difficult, and this investigation is probably best left to the specialist.

Treatment of low back pain
Management of acute low back pain and sciatica

While often due to a disc prolapse or intervertebral joint derangement, the possibilities of neoplastic or osteoporotic collapse of a vertebra must always be remembered, especially

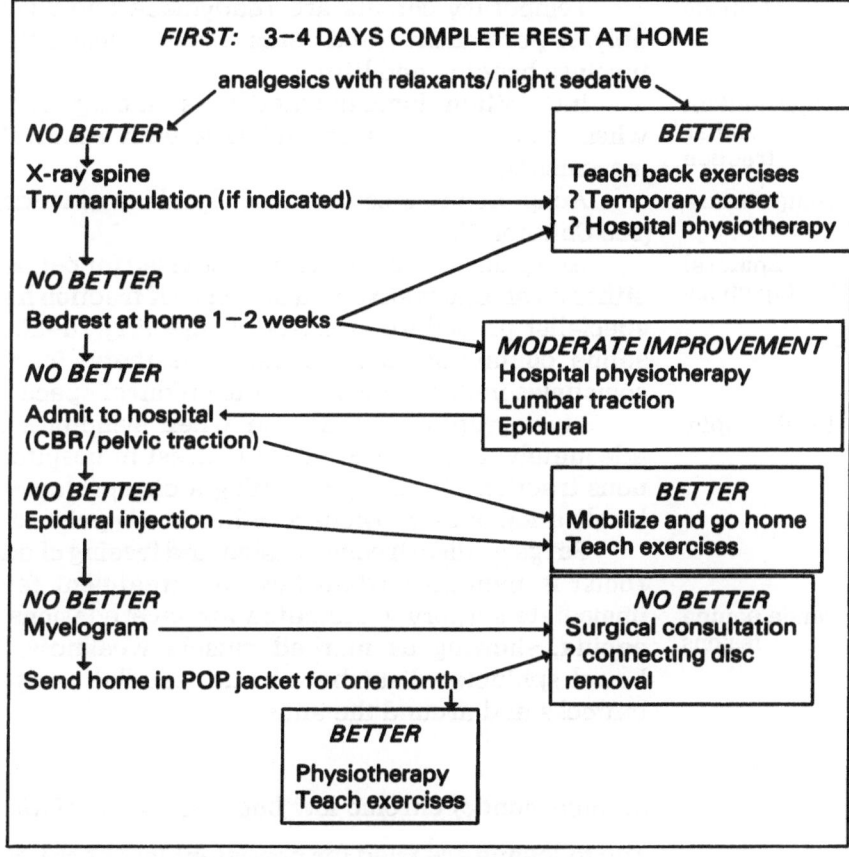

Figure 11.2   Management of acute low back pain and sciatica

in elderly patients. The management of disc lesions and osteoarthritis may be illustrated as shown in Figure 11.2.

Notes on the various treatments

Bedrest at home
: 'Bedrest' at home is not the same as complete bedrest in hospital – it is, of course, much less complete. Patients are often themselves amazed at the effect of a few days enforced rest in hospital.

Manipulation of lumbar spine
: Manipulation of the lumbar spine is indicated when acute pain due to a 'locked' intervertebral joint persists after a few days rest. It is useless in true sciatica, especially of insidious onset.

Back exercises
: Back exercises are usually simple extension exercises (see Chapter 5 and the reproduced handout of exercises for patients at end of this chapter – Table 11.1).

Corsets
: Temporary corsets are readymade and must fit comfortably. A permanent fitted corset may be desirable where work involves bending and lifting.

Intermittent lumbar traction
: Intermittent lumbar traction as an outpatient is indicated when there is persistent sciatica with relatively free back movements.

Acupuncture
: Acupuncture is sometimes helpful for minor degrees of pain (see Chapter 5).

Epidural injections
: An epidural injection may be advised for persistent sciatica, either as an alternative to traction or if traction has failed. This specialist procedure consists of injecting 20–50 ml of normal saline containing dilute local anaesthetic (corticosteroid is sometimes included also) into the epidural space.

Myelography
: Myelography is indicated when symptoms fail to settle adequately after 2 or 3 weeks bedrest in hospital with continuous traction. Besides confirming a disc prolapse it allows the localization of disc lesions at other levels prior to surgery.

Surgery (disc decompression and freeing of adherent nerve roots) is indicated when hospital treatment fails. However, immediate surgery is indicated for severe lesions of the cauda equina, showing as marked muscle weakness, bladder and bowel sphincter disturbance and 'saddle' analgesia over the buttocks and around the anus.

Cauda equina lesions

Management of chronic low back pain and sciatica

The following are tried for persistent low back pain, though not necessarily in the order given:

(1) Physiotherapy (heat and exercise therapy).
(2) Manipulations.
(3) Provision of a corset.
(4) Intermittent lumbar traction. } especially where
(5) Epidural injection. } sciatica is prominent
(6) Acupuncture – especially where the pain is referred (as opposed to true sciatica with root paraesthesia).

The following patient handout on exercises for low back pain (Table 11.1) describing simple exercises for low back pain has been found useful.

Table 11.1 Exercises for low back pain

Carry out the following exercises two or three times daily:
(two on your back, two lying on your stomach),

On your back
(1) Straight-leg raising, one leg at a time. Get legs as high as you can.
(2) With the knees bent, lift your bottom up until the back is straight, then lower your bottom. Repeat until tired.

On your stomach
(1) Straight-leg raising, as high as each will go without hurting too much.
(2) Clasp hands behind the back, lift the head and shoulders as high as you can go without hurting too much. Then lower and repeat.

Note: No exercise should be painful and any exercise which produces pain in the leg should be stopped immediately.

---

12 Pain syndromes of the upper limb

Causes of pain –Diagnosis and treatment of pain

Pain in the arm is a very common complaint. It is either brachial neuralgia –pain travelling down the whole arm usually due to a cervical disc lesion – or else localized pain in the shoulder, elbow wrist or hand. There may be a combination of these, for instance, pain referred from cervical spondylosis may summate with a tennis elbow, and perhaps also a carpal tunnel syndrome. This chapter's main message is that for adequate and effective treatment we must recognize *all* sites from which brachial pain is derived.

Causes of pain

Pain in the arm is usually derived from one or more of the following structures:

(1) Cervical spine (disc/spondylosis).
(2) Thoracic outlet.
(3) Shoulder (rotator cuff lesion/capsulitis).
(4) Elbow (tennis elbow/golfer's elbow/arthritis).
(5) Wrist (tenosynovitis/arthritis).
(6) Hand (arthritis/carpal tunnel syndrome).

Brachial neuralgia

Brachial neuralgia is usually due to cervical spondylosis or one or more disc lesions. The pain is of segmental distribution,

125

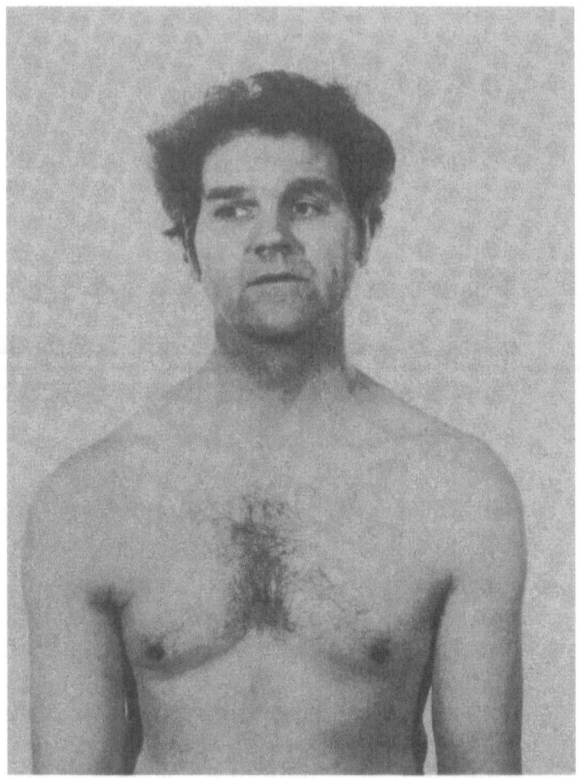

Figure 12.1

Marked drooping of the shoulder girdles, which together with fusion of the cervical vertebrae, comprises the Klippel–Fleil syndrome

according to the level involved, and is usually associated with paraesthesia in the same segment. A more vague type of referred pain, without paraesthesia or neurological signs, may also occur – this (but not true root pain) often responds to acupuncture. Sometimes brachial neuralgia due to compression of the brachial plexus nerve trunks in the thoracic outlet – there may be a cervical rib, but more often the cause is simply poor posture, with sagging shoulders and 'drooping shoulder-girdles (see Figure 12.1) – such cases often respond to simple postural training and shoulder-raising exercises. The pain and paraesthesia are typically in the medial side of the arm and little finger, as it is principally the lower trunk of the brachial plexus which is compressed, and in severe cases there are vasomotor symptoms due to subclavian artery compression as well.

Pain syndromes of the upper limb

Shoulder pain

Causes

In shoulder disorders the pain is felt in the upper arm, usually over the triceps, rather than around the shoulder itself. Anterior shoulder pain radiating down the biceps denotes bicipital tendinitis, which is a common precursor of capsulitis (frozen shoulder). The common causes of painful shoulders are:

(1) Rotator cuff lesions (inflammation or trauma of the common insertion of supraspinatus, infraspinatus and teres monor).
(2) Cervical spondylosis or disc (referred pain).
(3) Capsulitis (periarthritis, 'frozen shoulder').
(4) Polymyalgia rheumatica.

Less common causes of painful shoulder are fractures, dislocations, referred pain from the upper thoracic spine, osteoarthritis (rare in the shoulder, unlike the hip), severe carpal tunnel syndrome (pain referred up the arm), neuralgic amyotrophy ('shoulder-girdle neuritis', probably due to a virus attack on the cervical rami), and referred pain from the chest (such as apical lung carcinoma), heart (myocardial insufficiency) or gallbladder (acute cholecystitis).

Diagnosis

The clinical diagnosis of shoulder problems is based on (a) the site and referral of pain, and (b) whether the shoulder movements are restricted in most planes:

Rotator cuff lesions
Polymyalgia rheumatica   } Movements
Referred pain (from spine or viscera)   } not
                                  } limited

Capsulitis ('frozen shoulder' in its fully
developed form)   } Movements
Intra-articular lesions (arthritis, fractures, } limited
tumours)

Capsulitis of shoulder

In capsulitis of the shoulder, the movements are limited in all planes. In rotator cuff lesions there may be some degree of painful limitation of abduction, but careful examination shows that the movements are in fact almost full (though painful). In 'classical' supraspinatus lesions there is a painful arc on abduc-

127

The stiff
shoulder
X-rays

tion – movement is painful in the mid-arc, but on raising and lowering the arm. Radiographs of the shoulder in long-standing or recurrent rotator cuff lesions may show calcific deposits (the calcium salt is usually hydroxyapatite). Radiographs are normal in capsulitis, but nevertheless it is wise to X-ray the stiff, painful shoulder to exclude osteoarthritis (which, unlike the hip, is very uncommon in the shoulder) and rare conditions such as neoplasms which do crop up occasionally.

Treatment

Rotator cuff
lesion of
shoulder

Capsulitis of the shoulder and rotator cuff lesions are different clinical entities (though the latter may progress to become a frozen shoulder) and the treatment is different. A rotator cuff lesion, especially a clear-cut supraspinatus lesion, often – though not always – responds to a local steroid injection into the site of the lesion, that is, at the point of maximal tenderness, not the site of pain. This is followed by *gentle* physiotherapy – vigorous exercises in the acute stage can aggravate the condition. With regard to capsulitis, this goes through three stages (which last 9–12 months altogether) and the correct management of a frozen shoulder depends on the stage at which the patient is seen.

Stages of
shoulder
capsulitis

The stages of capsulitis and their treatment are as shown in Table 12.1 below.

Table 12.1   The stages of capsulitis and their treatment

Stage I: acute stage	pain + +, movements ↡↡ Try pericapsular injection of steroid, anti-inflammatory drugs. Rest the arm, do not exercise. Pain should be relieved but movements will remain limited.
Stage II: subacute stage	pain +, Movements ↡↡ Treat expectantly. A further steroid injection can be tried. Very gentle physiotherapy may be introduced.
Stage III: chronic stage	no pain (or only minimal discomfort) at rest or on movement. Movements ↡↡ and later improve. Physiotherapy, home exercises. Refer to rheumatologist for consideration of manipulation under anaesthesia if progress is slow.

Elbow pain

Tennis or golfer's elbow

This is usually due to one of the enthesopathies, tennis elbow (lateral epicondylitis) or golfer's elbow (medial epicondylitis). Occasionally there is slight synovitis and rheumatoid or osteo-arthritis or gout is found to be the cause. Tennis and golfer's elbow usually respond to local steroid injections in the site of maximal tenderness at the common extensor/flexor origin followed by a few weeks rest to allow the lesion to heal. Resting the arm is important – failure to respond often means that the arm has not been rested due to continuation of the sport or repetitive activity at work. Another reason for failure is that there is an underlying condition – such as cervical spondylosis, osteoarthritis of the elbow or atypical gout – to which the epi-condylitis is 'secondary'. These conditions may not be obvious and their investigation often falls to the rheumatologist. Physio-therapy (massage or ultrasound) though often prescribed for tennis elbow is not usually helpful except in very chronic cases where there is thickening of the common extensor or flexor origin due to adhesions. Very occasionally surgery is required, but since most tennis elbows eventually resolve within 2–3 years, orthopaedic surgeons are not keen to operate except under special circumstances such as when severe pain ser-iously interferes with work.

Wrist pain

This is either 'referred' pain from the cervical spine, or comes from tenosynovitis of one of the related tendons, such as the flexor tendons at the front of the wrist, or is due to arthritis of the wrist – usually rheumatoid arthritis, as osteoarthritis of the wrist is uncommon (unless there has been an antecedent frac-ture or other injury). The basis of treatment is splinting and local steroid injections (plus, of course, management of the under-lying disease such as rheumatoid arthritis).

Pain in the fingers and hands

Pain in the fingers and hands is usually due to *arthritis*, where there is joint swelling, or else *tenosynovitis* of the flexor or extensor tendons (which itself may be due to rheumatoid arth-ritis). The most common cause of pain and paraesthesia in the hands, usually worse at night, is the *carpal tunnel syndrome* which is due to some form of entrapment of the median nerve at

129

Referral for
electro-
diagnosis

the front of the wrist. The pressure on the nerve may be due to fluid retention (as in pregnancy or the menopause), a displaced Colles fracture, tenosynovitis, or myxoedema; there are other causes, but usually the condition is idiopathic. In all but the mildest cases of the carpal tunnel syndrome referral for electro-diagnosis is advisable, for two reasons: to corroborate the diagnosis, and to assess the severity of the condition which is indicated by the increase of latency of median nerve condition and reduction of its terminal conduction velocity. Mild cases of the carpal tunnel syndrome often respond to diuretics, splinting, or injection of steroid into the carpal tunnel. Severe cases, and many only moderately severe cases, usually require surgical decompression of the median nerve.

Diagnosis and treatment of pain

We are now in a position to summarize the detailed investigation of a patient presenting with pain in the arm. The following flowchart (Table 12.2) indicates the sequence of examination, investigations and treatment.

Table 12.2 Examination, investigation and treatment of arm pain

Examine patient starting from the neck and working downwards

EXAMINE CERVICAL SPINE

Neck movements, neurological examination of arms local tenderness on cervical spine ↓

EXAMINE THORACIC OUTLET

Note shoulder posture, palpate for cervical rib, auscultate for supraclavicular bruit (suggests brachial artery aneurysm), note vasomotor symptoms in hands,

X-ray for cervical rib ↓

EXAMINE SHOULDERS

Note muscle wasting, movements, site of local tenderness

X-ray if indicated ↓

EXAMINE ELBOWS

Note epicondylar and joint tenderness, any synovial swelling, elicit Mills' sign (pain on resisted extension in tennis elbow), note any limitation of movements (arthritis)
↓
EXAMINE WRISTS AND HANDS

Note joint swelling, tenderness, tenosynovitis

Note wasting, hypalgesia in median nerve distribution in carpal tunnel syndrome: confirm by electrodiagnosis.

130

It must again be stressed that there may be *lesions at several levels*, each requiring individual treatment. For example, the following scheme might represent correct treatment of such a case (Table 12.3).

Table 12.3   A 'multilevel' case of arm pain

First visit	course of intermittent cervical traction; teach shoulder-raising exercises ↓
Second visit	inject ('secondary') tennis elbow; inject rotator cuff lesion of shoulder ↓
Third visit	median nerve conduction tests confirm carpal tunnel syndrome; inject carpal tunnel with steroid
Fourth visit	carpal tunnel syndrome responds only temporarily to steroid injection; refer for surgical decompression

13 Pain syndromes of the lower limb

Causes of pain – Diagnosis and treatment of pain – Causes of painful feet

Pain in the leg, like arm pain, comes from one or more individual structures in the lower limb, or else it is referred (usually from the spine).

Causes of pain

Pain in the leg is usually derived from one (or more than one) of the following structures (the commonest disorders are given in brackets).

(1) Lumbar spine (disc/spondylosis).
(2) Hip (osteoarthritis).
(3) Knee (arthritis/ligamentous strain or internal derangement).
(4) Ankle and foot (arthritis/strain or sprain).
(5) Arterial insufficiency (intermittent claudication).
(6) Venous insufficiency or inflammation (thrombophlebitis).

Sciatica

Sciatica is of course the name given to pain radiating down the leg from a lumbar spine lesion. True sciatica is segmental nerve pain associated with paraesthesiae, and there is usually some objective evidence of lumbar nerve-root pressure, such as a

Neurogenic
claudication

diminished reflex. However, as in the arm a less well-defined and less severe *referred pain* may occur. This is not accompanied by paraesthesia or objective neurological signs and does not necessarily denote a prolapsed disc. Sciatica may be claudicating in nature. This *'neurogenic claudication'* may be due to a prolapsed lumbar disc and is sometimes associated with spinal stenosis. It occasionally responds to outpatient treatment of simple spinal traction, but severe cases may require surgical treatment and this is particularly the case where there is significant spinal stenosis.

Diagnosis and treatment of pain

The treatment of sciatica due to a prolapsed lumbar disc is described in Chapter 11.

Hip pain

Osteoarthritis
of hips

Pain in the hip region is often referred from the lumbar spine and not due to pathology in the hip joint. Here the physician may be deceived by apparent restriction of hip movements due to 'secondary' muscle spasm. In osteoarthritis of the hip pain is aggravated by weight bearing, and movements are definitely restricted in more than one direction; radiographs prove the diagnosis, show the type and severity of the arthritis, and predisposing factors such as congenital dislocation of the hip or old injury. With regard to treatment of osteoarthritis of the hip, it must be clearly understood by both the doctor and patient that conservative treatment is rarely satisfactory. Anti-inflammatory drugs may help, but except in very early cases, physiotherapy is usually a waste of time, though occasionally exercises in the hydrotherapy pool provide temporary relief.

Surgery for
O.A. hip

Surgery (osteotomy or total replacement) is usually required at some stage and prosthetic replacement is often highly successful in relieving pain and restoring movements.

Knee pain

Osteoarthritis
of the knees

Pain in the knee may be referred from the hip (usually to the medial side). Unfortunately osteoarthritis can begin in quite young people, even in the early twenties, when physical signs may be minimal and the X-ray shows no abnormality. Mild cases are often well managed with local steroids and physiotherapy (see Chapter 5), but severe osteoarthritis may be a source of

134

Surgery for
O.A. knees

Medial
ligament
strain

Internal
derangements
of the knee

severe debility due perhaps to valgus or varus deformities needing surgical treatment. Occasionally prosthetic replacement of
the knee is possible. Again, symptoms due to osteoarthritis
located to the patellofemoral joint is relieved by patellectomy, a
simple operation which is particularly useful in older patients.
A very common cause of pain in the medial side of the knee is
medial ligament strain which may be due to simple trauma or
secondary to underlying osteoarthritis. It usually responds to a
local steroid injection. *Internal derangements of the knee*,
mainly involving the menisci ('cartilages'), are usually thought
of as due to trauma in young men, but a similar picture may
occur due to degenerative lesions of the menisci as part of osteoarthritis in middle-aged or elderly patients.

Heel pain

Achilles
tendinitis

Plantar
fasciitis

Pain in the heel usually relates to either Achilles tendinitis (pain,
tenderness and slight swelling of the Achilles tendon at the back
of the heel, which is usually traumatic or 'idiopathic' but
occasionally turns out to be a feature of rheumatoid disease or
seronegative arthritis) or plantar fasciitis (pain and tenderness
under the heel – an enthesopathy of the plantar fascia). Less
common causes of heel pain include Paget's disease of bone,
stress fractures and osteochondritis of the calcaneum.

Ankle pain

Sprained
ankle

Pain in the ankle usually means a strain or sprain, or perhaps
some form of arthritis. Osteoarthritis of the ankle is often
secondary to previous trauma which may be repetitive, such as
'footballer's ankle', or a single traumatic incident such as a
Pott's fracture. Sprains usually involve the lateral ligament of
the ankle. Acute sprains should be treated with ice applications,
ultrasound, sometimes a steroid injection into the ligament.
Chronic sprains require rather long courses of physiotherapy,
and it is important to correct abnormal mechanics, such as pes
planus (see below).

Causes of painful feet

The principal causes are:

(1) Deformities, such as severe pes planus.
(2) Osteoarthritis, rheumatoid arthritis or gout.

(3) Vascular disorders affecting the feet – intermittent claudication due to arteriosclerosis or Buerger's disease.

(4) Nerve compression – interdigital neuroma, or tarsal tunnel syndrome.

Pes planus

Various degrees of flat feet (pes planus) are, of course, present very often. When this is severe it may not only be responsible for foot discomfort, but it may throw abnormal strains upwards, and cause painful conditions of the hips, knees and even the back. One or both arches of the feet may be affected. Dropping of the anterior (metatarsal) arches sometimes causes anterior foot pain, but may be an early feature of rheumatoid arthritis as shown by tenderness of the lateral metatarsophalangeal joints. Here anterior (transverse) arch supports are important. The full flat-foot syndrome also includes dropping of the longitudinal arches. It is painful when the foot is stiff, either due to arthritis or occasionally, in young patients, due to a congenital abnormality such as vertical talus

Treatment of flat feet

or congenital bar. Here mobilization of the foot by exercises, often helped by wax therapy, and strengthening of the muscles supporting the arches by faradic foot baths and exercises, as well as provision of insoles incorporating both valgus and anterior arch supports, are important.

Morton's metatarsalgia

Finally, nerve entrapment syndromes in the feet include the occasional interdigital neuroma, usually formed by compression of an interdigital nerve between the metatarsal heads with pain shooting into the toes (Morton's metatarsalgia). This usually requires surgical removal. In the tarsal tunnel

Tarsal tunnel syndrome

syndrome, analogous to the carpal tunnel syndrome at the wrist, the posterior tibial nerve is compressed by the flexor retinaculum at the medial side of the ankle. As in the carpal tunnel syndrome, this condition should be confirmed, and its severity established, by testing posterior tibial nerve conductions. It may be relieved by a local steroid injection, but, just as in the carpal tunnel syndrome, surgical release of the flexor retinaculum may be required for complete relief of symptoms.

Appendix

Glossary of rheumatic disorders

Achilles tendinitis
Pain and sometimes swelling of Achilles tendons ('heel cords'); may be traumatic, or secondary to underlying inflammatory arthritis (such as Reiter's disease)

Acromegalic arthritis
Articular cartilage hypertrophy; enlarged wrists: compression of median nerves in carpal tunnels; synovial joints may be painful and enlarged; backache: enlarged vertebrae, calcified intervertebral discs

Acromioclavicular arthritis
Pain and swelling due to osteoarthritis/mild subluxation of acromioclavicular joints

Agammaglobinaemia arthritis
See: hypogammaglobinaemia

Amyloid joint disease
Amyloid infiltration of joints, tendons and carpal tunnels; in association with multiple myeloma, or secondary to severe rheumatoid disease

Ankylosing hyperostosis (Forestier's disease)
Backache: large osteophytes bridging vertebrae and forming anterior band simulating ankylosing spondylitis, but sacroiliac joints normal; some patients are diabetic or pre-diabetic.

Ankylosing spondylitis
Backache: mainly young adult males; marked hereditary factors – histocompatibility antigen HLA-B27 present in over 90% of patients; limited back movements in all planes, limited chest expansion; typical radiological changes in

spine and sacroiliac joints; hips and shoulders often affected, rarely small joints; anterior uveitis (common), specific aortic lesion (rare)

Aortic arch syndrome

See Pulseless disease

Atrophic polychondritis

See: Relapsing polychondritis

Behçet's syndrome

Episodic iritis and painful orogenital ulceration; occasional thrombophlebitis, neurological and other manifestations; arthritis in over 50% of cases, chronic or episodic

Bicipital tendinitis

Non-specific inflammation of tendon of long head of biceps, either at anterior aspect of shoulder or at its insertion in cubital fossa

Brachial neuralgia

See Neuralgia

Brucella arthritis

Arthralgia or backache (due to spondylitis) in brucellosis; occasionally, chronic destructive changes due to joint or spine infection

Bursitis

Swelling or effusions into bursae; traumatic or secondary to rheumatoid arthritis or gout

Caplan's syndrome (rheumatoid pneumoconiosis)

Characteristic radiological appearance of lungs in patients with pneumoconiosis who develop rheumatoid disease; multiple nodules on fibrotic background

Capsulitis of shoulder (periarthritis, frozen shoulder)

Inflammation and fibrosis of shoulder-joint capsule and surrounding tissues; shoulder initially painful and stiff, later pain subsides but stiffness persists for months; usually idiopathic, but predisposing causes include trauma, myocardial infarction, cervical spondylosis

Carpal tunnel syndrome

Pain and paraesthesiae in median nerve distribution of hand due to compression of nerve in carpal tunnel; usually no obvious cause, occasionally oedema, tenosynovitis, etc. compresses nerve; occasionally, wasting of thenar eminence; median nerve conduction latency increased

Cervical disc lesion/spondylosis

Lateral disc herniation/osteoarthritis of cervical spine;

neck pain and stiffness; segmental pain and paraesthesia in arm and hand; occasionally, segmental wasting of hand muscles, cord pressure causing cervical myelopathy), fainting attacks due to vertebrobasilar insufficiency.

Charcot's joints (neuropathic arthritis)

In certain lower motor neurone diseases, especially tabes, diabetes, syringomyelia and polyneuritis; joints enlarged, usually painless, sometimes unstable

Chondrocalcinosis

Crystal deposition in joints of soft tissues (urate, apatite or pyrophosphate crystals); recurrent attacks of pain (pseudogout), effusions or chronic arthritis

Chondromalacia patellae

Premature degeneration of patellar cartilage; recurrent pain/slight swelling of knees

Colitic arthritis

See Enteropathic arthritis

Crohn's disease

See: Enteropathic arthritis

Crystal deposition disease

See: Chondrocalcinosis

Dermatomyositis

Systemic connective tissue disorder characterized by myositis and skin lesions especially in the elderly; sometimes secondary to (latent) malignant neoplasm; proximal muscles weak, may be painful; serum muscle enzymes raised; rashes: heliotrope eruption on face, circumorbital oedema, violaceous rash on knuckles; arthralgia often occurs

Disc lesions

See under Cervical, Thoracic and Lumbar disc lesions

Enteropathic arthritis

Peripheral arthritis and sacroiliitis associated with ulcerative colitis, Crohn's disease or Whipple's disease (q.v.); episodic seronegative arthritis affecting mainly lower limb joints, flaring with activity of intestinal disease; backache due to sacroiliitis (does not parallel intestinal disease)

Epicondylitis

See: Tennis elbow, and Golfer's elbow

Erythema nodosum, arthritis with

Painful bluish papulonodular rash on legs; arthralgia, usually lower limbs, for a few weeks or months; most cases are associated with pulmonary sarcoid (bilateral hilar adenopathy), occasionally focal streptococcal infections, enteropathic arthritis or Behçet's disease.

Felty's syndrome

Rheumatoid arthritis with hypersplenism: splenomegaly, leukopenia, thrombocytopenia; recurrent infections, due to poor neutrophil chemotaxis

Fibrositis

Lay term for pain due to muscle spasm, often in the spine; it usually represents referred pain from spinal conditions such as spondylosis

Frozen shoulder

See: Capsulitis

Giant cell arteritis

See: Temporal arteritis

Golfer's elbow

Epicondylitis (a form of enthesopathy) at medial side of elbow, involving common flexor origin from medial epicondyle of humerus

Gout

A form of acute synovitis due to deposition of urate crystals, in patients (mainly males) who have metabolic error leading to high serum urate levels; strong familial tendency; classical attacks of severe pain in metatarsophalangeal joint of big toe spreading up the foot; occasionally, polyarticular attacks; when chronic: urate deposits lead to tophi formation, chronic arthritis and renal failure; secondary gout: due to excess urate production (as in polycythaemia vera) or decreased urate excretion (as in chronic renal failure); raised serum uric acid, synovial fluid contains needle-shaped urate cyrstals.

Haemarthrosis

Bleeding into a synovial joint causing severe pain and swelling (as in haemophilia) and not infrequently in osteoarthritic joints in elderly patients

Haemophilic arthritis

Acute haemarthroses due to haemorrhages into joints in haemophilia and other haemorrhagic disorders; secondary osteoarthritis often supervenes

Henoch–Schonlein purpura

Acute arthritis, usually of knees or ankles, with petechial

rash particularly on buttocks, usually in children; abdominal pain and melaena may occur; haematuria, nephritis in some cases

Hydrarthrosis, intermittent

Periodic effusions into large joints, especially knees; aetiology uncertain – no connection with rheumatoid disease

Hypermobility syndrome

Local or generalized pain syndromes due to strain on ligaments in hypermobile joints; effusions may occur, eventually osteoarthritis; sometimes hereditary (as in Marfan's syndrome) or metabolic (such as homocystinuria); backache due to 'loose back syndrome' often associated with generalized hypermobility

Hyperparathyroidism

Abnormal calcium metabolism may lead to spinal osteoporosis, metastatic calcification or pyrophosphate arthropathy (q.v.); synovitis associated with softening of para-articular bone

Hypertrophic osteoarthropathy

Arthropathy, finger clubbing and periostitis usually associated with malignant tumour (especially bronchogenic carcinoma)

Hypogammaglobinaemia, arthritis with

Seronegative arthritis resembling rheumatoid in patients with low or absent gammaglobulin and immunoglobulin G; congenital and acquired varieties; mainly large joints involved, often asymmetrical; recurrent respiratory tract infections

Hypothyroidism

Muscular rheumatism or arthralgia may occur; symptoms respond to thyroid replacement; carpal tunnel syndrome is common

Infective arthritis

See: Septic arthritis

Intermittent hydrarthrosis

See: Hydrarthrosis, intermittent

Jaccoud syndrome (chronic secondary polyarthritis)

Tendon lesions of hands due to fibrosis, hand deformities (ulnar deviation) following recurrent attacks of rheumatic fever

Juvenile chronic arthritis
   Arthritis in children (see Still's disease)

Leukaemic arthritis
   Arthritis in acute leukaemia in children; secondary gout may occur; arthritis in chronic leukaemia of adults

Lumbar disc lesions/spondylosis
   Traumatic or degenerative lesions of vertebrae and inter-vertebral discs; low back pain with or without sciatica in lateral disc prolapse, paraesthesiae in root distribution (commonly L_5–S_1); occasionally, segmental muscle weakness and wasting; limited straight leg raising (lower lumbar lesions), positive femoral nerve stretch (upper lumbar lesions); cauda equina lesions: weakness, bladder and bowel sphincter disturbance, perianal analgesia

Lupus erythematosis
   See: Systemic lupus erythematosus (SLE)

Mixed connective tissue disease
   Combination of various systemic connective tissue diseases, such as rheumatoid arthritis, systemic sclerosis and SLE, overlapping in the same patient. ANA-positive but DNA-binding negative and antiRNA antibodies positive; prognosis said to be good but many cases later 'polarize' to become a more definite systemic connective tissue disorder with its appropriate prognosis

Morton's metatarsalgia
   Pain between toes, said to be due to neurofibroma of anastomosing plantar digital nerves

Myelomatosis (multiple myeloma)
   Monoclonal gammopathy due to excess plasma cells, with paraprotein deposition in bone and soft tissues; electro-phoresis shows paraprotein (dense abnormal band); back pain due to vertebral involvement; peripheral arthropathy from secondary amyloid deposition; Bence-Jones protein-uria in some cases; carpal tunnel syndrome, secondary gout, hypercalcaemia and renal failure may occur

Myxoedema
   See: Hypothyroidism

Neuralgia, brachial
   Pain radiating down arm usually with paraesthesia of root distribution; commonly due to nerve-root involvement in cervical spondylosis or disc lesion

Neuropathic arthritis
See: Charcot joints

Ochronotic arthropathy (ochronosis)
Hereditary arthropathy due to disorder of tyrosine metabolism: accumulation of homogentisic acid in cartilage; alcaptonuria (urine goes black on standing due to homogentisic acid; spine: calcification of intervertebral discs, limited movements; large joints (knees and shoulders) painful and stiff; ear and nose cartilages appear brown

Osteitis condensans ilii
Radiological appearance of para-articular sclerosis of ilial side of sacroiliac joints without erosions or narrowing of the joints; a disputed cause of low back pain, especially in females

Osteoarthritis (osteoarthrosis)
Degenerative joint disease; involvement of certain joints (such as TIP joints of fingers, MTP joints of big toes) characteristic; joints stiff, moderately painful, movements limited; effusions in large joints sometimes due to crystal deposition; deformities mainly due to cartilage loss, such as genu valgum; acute synovitis and attacks of pain (probably due to calcium apatite deposition) may occur

Osteochondritis
Non-specific inflammation of bone and cartilage in young people often affecting epiphyses of growing bones; examples: Perthes disease (osteochondritis of femoral head), Schuermann's disease (vertebrae), Osgood–Schlatter's disease (tibial tubercle)

Paget's disease of bone
Bone absorption with concurrent new bone formation; asymptomatic lesions (seen on X-ray) common; back and limb pains are common and deformity may occur; skull large, when involved; raised serum alkaline phosphatase (acid phosphatase normal) in active disease; complications: osteoarthritis of associated joints, osteogenic sarcoma

Palindromic rheumatism
Episodic arthritis or arthralgia; joint pain is often very severe, swelling slight or absent; intervals between attacks almost symptom free; many patients later develop rheumatoid arthritis

Panniculitis

Painful localized fat deposits, often around knees in menopausal women; pain is often confused with that due to
associated osteoarthritis.

Plantar fasciitis

Commonest cause of pain under the heel: an enthesopathy
(tenoperiostitis of attachment of plantar fascia to inferior
surface of calcaneum); a 'simple spur' is commonly seen in
X-ray; rarely, a 'compound spur' indicating inflammation
and periosteal reaction secondary to ankylosing spondylitis, Reiter's disease or other seronegative spondarthritis

Polyarteritis (polyarteritis nodosa)

Systemic connective tissue disorder involving arteries;
necrotizing arteritis of all three coats, Australia antigen
(hepatitis B) occasionally present; protein manifestations:
arthralgia, fever, peripheral neuropathy, renal disease,
lung disease, coronary artery disease, peripheral neuropathy, abdominal pain and intestinal infarction; negative
tests for rheumatoid factor (unless polyarteritis is secondary to rheumatoid disease)

Polymyalgia rheumatica

Syndrome of central joint pain, morning stiffness and high
ESR in the elderly. Some cases due to cranial arteritis, some
idiopathic, some are prodromal rheumatoid arthritis and
some herald malignancy or myelomatosis

Polymyositis

Polymyositis is dermatomyositis (q.v.) without skin lesions;
secondary polymyositis may occur in any systemic connective tissue disorder, such as polyarteritis, systemic sclerosis, mixed connective tissue disease and systemic lupus

Pseudogout

See: Chondrocalcinosis

Psoriatic arthritis

Atypical seronegative arthritis associated with psoriasis
(or psoriasis in a close relative); 10% of psoriatic patients
with psoriasis will develop psoriatic arthritis

Four types: (a) indeterminate, resembling rheumatoid
arthritis, (b) classical, characterized by erosions of terminal interphalangeal joints, (c) mutilating, with osteolysis
and gross deformities of hands and feet, (d) spondylitic,
resembling ankylosing spondylitis.

Special features include 'sausage toes' (inflammation of
joints and soft tissues), bony ankylosis, sacroiliitis, spondylitis, paravertebral ligamentous ossification

Pulseless disease (aortic arch syndrome or Takayusu's disease)
variety of arteritis affecting branches of aortic arch; absent upper limb pulses, cerebral ischaemia, involvement of retinal arteries

Pyrophosphate arthropathy
See: Chondrocalcinosis

de Quervain's disease
Common form of tenosynovitis affecting flexor sheath of abductor pollicis longus and extensor pollicis brevis at radial side of the wrist

Reiter's disease
Seronegative spondarthritis (HLA-B27 often present) associated with non-specific urethritis and conjunctivitis, usually post-venereal; lower limb large joints usually affected; tenosynovitis and Achilles tendinitis common; sacroiliitis develops in many cases (occasionally spondylitis); other occasional features: balanitis, buccal ulceration, keratoderma blennorhagica

Relapsing polychondritis
Rare disorder in which cartilage degenerates and becomes inflamed; polyarthritis may occur, ears and nose 'flop'

Rheumatic fever
Polyarthritis, carditis and fever in children and young adults following focal infection with beta-haemolytic streptococcus; sore throat followed by migratory polyarthritis of large joints; carditis often followed by permanent valvular damage; Jaccoud's syndrome (q.v.) rarely follows repeated attacks; occasionally, painful subcutaneous 'rheumatic nodules' (smaller than rheumatoid nodules), erythema nodosum or erythema marginatum

Rheumatoid arthritis
Inflammatory, usually seropositive polyarthritis (occasionally monarthritis or pauciarthritis); classically symmetrical with erosion of joints and subsequent deformity; joints are painful, stiff, tender and swollen due to synovial hypertrophy or effusion, later articular cartilage is eroded; soft tissue involvement includes subcutaneous nodules, tenosynovitis, bursitis; extra-articular lesions in some cases: myopathy, neuropathy, vasculitis, eye lesions, pulmonary lesions; anaemia common and proportional to disease

activity; sheep cell agglutination and latex tests for rheumatoid factor positive in 80% of adult cases.

Rotator cuff syndrome
See: Supraspinatus tendinitis

Rubella arthritis
Arthralgia or joint effusions following rubella infection,
usually a few days after the rash or 2–4 weeks after rubella
vaccination; carpal tunnel syndrome common; joint
symptoms subside after some weeks.

Sacroiliitis
Non-specific inflammation of sacroiliac joints causing low
backache in ankylosing spondylitis and other varieties of
seronegative spondarthritis; X-rays show widening,
irregularity or erosions of sacroiliac joints

Sarcoid arthritis
Transient polyarthritis, usually with erythema nodosum
(q.v.); rarely, chronic asymmetrical joint swelling due to
sarcoid involvement of synovial membrane

Sciatica
Pain radiating down one or both legs, usually due to prolapse of lumbar intervertebral disc; paraesthesiae in corresponding segments often accompanies sciatic pain

Scleroderma
See: Systemic sclerosis

Septic arthritis
Severe arthritis, usually monarticular, following pyogenic
infection which is either haematogenous or due to local
infection of joint; joint is very painful and tender, often red
and hot; synovial fluid purulent with marked rise in white
cell count, organisms may be cultured

Shoulder–hand syndrome
Capsulitis of shoulder (q.v.) associated with pain, swelling
and vasomotor disturbance of ipsilateral hand in early
stages; later hand becomes atrophic, with patchy osteoporosis on X-ray (a form of algodystrophy)

Sjogren's syndrome
Rheumatoid arthritis (or other systemic connective tissue
disease) with keratoconjunctivitis sicca; exocrine glands
involved causing xerostomia, swollen parotid glands, nasal
dryness, atrophic vaginitis

Spondylitis
See: Ankylosing spondylitis. (*NB: do not* confuse with
spondylosis)

Spondylosis

Osteoarthritis of spine (see cervical spondylosis, lumbar spondylosis)

Still's disease

One variety of juvenile chronic arthritis (JCA); polyarthritis in some ways resembling rheumatoid arthritis, together with systemic features; arthritis particularly involves wrists and cervical spine at an early stage; seronegative, no subcutaneous nodules; growth stunting and epiphyseal disturbances common; in classical acute cases: pyrexia, maculopapular rash, lymphadenopathy, occasional splenomegaly; severe iritis is not uncommon, especially in the pauciarticular type of JCA.

Supraspinatus tendinitis

'Painful arc syndrome' – common cause of painful shoulder, due to non-specific inflammation of rotator cuff (common insertion of supraspinatus, infraspinatus and teres minor into greater tuberosity of humerus); often traumatic, may be idiopathic (degenerative); severe or recurrent cases may be associated with calcific (apatite) deposits

Systemic lupus erythematosus (SLE)

Connective tissue disorder characterized by lesions due to fibrinoid degeneration of walls of blood vessels and deposition of immune complexes; arthritis or arthralgia in all cases, but joint destruction and deformity is not common; characteristic rash in butterfly area of face; prognosis is poor, death usually due to renal involvement or cerebral involvement (in those without renal disease); other features include fever, cardiorenal disease, serositis, hepatomegaly and splenomegaly, blood dyscrasias, anaemia, neutropenia, thrombocytopenia, haemolytic anaemia; wide variety of immunological disorders include positive antinuclear antibodies, raised DNA-binding, LE cells in peripheral blood

Systemic sclerosis

Connective tissue disorder characterized by thickened skin and subcutaneous tissues due to increase in dermal collagen and atrophy of epidermia; skin shiny, thick, later ulcerated, occasionally telangiectatic; finger contractures due to dermal fibrosis, subcutaneous calcinosis; arthritis (seropositive or seronegative) of small joints is common and often difficult to distinguish from coexistent rheumatoid arthritis; dysphagia due to oesophageal fibrosis (shown by barium swallow) is characteristic; occasional features: myopathy, malabsorption due to gut involvement, pulmonary fibrosis, cardiac conduction defects, renal involvement causing malignant hypertension

Takayusu's disease
See: Pulseless disease

Tennis elbow
Non-specific inflammation of common extensor origin at the lateral epicondyle of the humerus (enthesopathy); commonest cause of pain in the elbow

Tenosynovitis
Non-specific inflammation of a tendon sheath (primary or secondary to inflammatory polyarthritis)

Tietze's syndrome
Attacks of pain, tenderness and swelling of costosternal joints; often self-limiting, subsiding within a year

Traumatic arthritis
Synovitis or arthralgia following trauma to joint; sudden onset of monarticular swelling of a normal or previously arthritic joint

Tuberculous arthritis
Monarticular arthritis due to infection by *Mycobacterium tuberculosis*; joint pain with marked wasting of adjacent muscles and swelling, with shiny, bluish overlying skin; back pain and subsequent deformities due to vertebral involvement; cold abscesses (paravertebral, for example).

Ulcerative colitis, arthritis with
See: Enteropathic arthritis

Wegener's granulomatosus
Necrotizing lesion of nasal cartilages together with widespread polyarteritis

Whipple's disease
Probably bacterial infection of intestinal mucosa and fat, causing malabsorption, lymphadenopathy and a form of episodic seronegative spondarthritis

Wilson's disease
Hepatolenticular degeneration due to copper accumulation in tissues, the various manifestations relating principally to liver and nervous system disorder; Kayser–Fleischer rings in cornea; premature osteoarthritis and joint hypermobility in some patients

Further reading

General textbooks of rheumatology

Scott, J. (ed.) (1980). *Copeman's Textbook of the Rheumatic Diseases, 6th Ed.* (Edinburgh: Churchill Livingstone). A large, comprehensive text, for selected rather than general reading

Mason, and Currey, (1980). *An Introduction to Clinical Rheumatology, 3rd Ed.* (London: Pitman). A small, compact book written for medical students, inclined to be theoretical rather than practical in its outlook

Golding, D., (19–). *Synopsis of the Rheumatic Diseases, 4th Ed.* (Bristol: J. Wright & Sons) (In preparation). A small, condensed text

Books related to management

Golding, D. (ed.) (1979). *Concise Management of the Common Rheumatic Disorders* (Bristol: J. Wright & Sons). Companion to *Synopsis*, emphasizing practical treatment

Hart, (ed.) (1978). *Drug Treatment of the Rheumatic Diseases* (Sydney: Adis Press). Useful information about all aspects of drug therapy

Hollingsworth, (1978). *Management of Rheumatoid Arthritis and its Complications* (Year Book Medical Publishers, Inc.) Detailed up-to-date management of all aspects of the disease

Index

153

Problems in arthritis and rheumatism